Brain Games

Richard B. Fisher

Brain Games

134 Original Scientific Games
That Reveal How Your Mind Works

SCHOCKEN BOOKS · NEW YORK

First American edition published by Schocken Books 1982
10 9 8 7 6 5 4 3 2 1   82 83 84 85
Copyright © Richard B. Fisher 1981
Published by agreement with Fontana Paperbacks, London

Library of Congress Cataloging in Publication Data
Fisher, Richard B.
    Brain games. 134 Original scientific games that
reveal how your mind works.
    1. Brain. 2. Educational games. I. Title.
QP376.F518   1982   793.7   81–84110
                                     AACR2

Manufactured in the United States of America
ISBN 0–8052–3800–X (hardback)
    0–8052–0707–4 (paperback)

Contents

Foreword

The games in this book are designed to entertain. Yet most of them were originally experiments conducted by research workers in their own laboratories. Indeed, it is far more difficult to design an experiment capable of answering a relevant question than it is to carry it out. I am grateful to the experimenters and indebted both to them and to other writers who have described the how as well as the why. Acknowledgements for individual games appear in the References at the end of the book.

Brain Games puts you in the shoes of a research scientist opening up new avenues of knowledge. In the process of playing the games, I hope you will also discover your own brain.

All the games in this book are easy. None of them requires any special training. As the list (p. 6) shows, even the necessary props and materials can be found in your own home. Many of the games need the help of a friend, occasionally more than one, and there is no reason why some of the games should not be fun at a party.

In most, the directions are very short. If the results you get are not those described, try again. In any case, do not allow a short-fall to spoil your enjoyment. Some of the games depend on your own background and personality, and the results may be variable. The important thing is that you see the point behind each game.

You will need a pen or pencil and paper for many of the games. A complete list of the other props and materials required is as follows:

blotter pad
books, about 3 doz. assorted
bookshelves, 2
bowls for water, 3
cellophane, 3 sheets (red,
  blue, green)
coffee or tea
coloured paper squares, 2
  inch
comfortable chair
electric razor
flashlights, 3
foot rule or equivalent
glasses or vases, 2
lamps, table or standard, 2

metronome (if available)
mirror, hand or wall
pictures from magazines or
  papers, 120–150
radio or record player,
  separate volume control
spoons, 2
stop watch (if available)
stove, gas, not
  automatic
string
toothpicks
washing machine
watch, wrist or pocket

Now, play on!

Brain Games

1 Personality

I

Game 1.1: Answer the following questions quickly, yes or no. Write down your answers, Y for yes and N for no:

1 Do you often wish for more excitement in your life?
2 Are you often late for appointments?
3 Are you impatient with fact-finding by others when you have made up your mind about something?
4 Do you prefer phoning to writing letters?
5 Do you often say things without thinking?
6 Are you generous with money?
7 Are you impatient with detailed directions when you think you see the point?
8 Do you accept the adage, 'He who hesitates is lost'?
9 Are you an organizer, a doer or an activist?
10 Do you get excited when you watch competitive sports?
11 Are you willing to 'have a go' even when you have no experience of the task?
12 Do you like to go out a lot?
13 Do you remember the faces of people you have met casually?
14 Do you consider that you control your own destiny?
15 Are you always in a hurry?
16 Do you often get ideas for new projects you want to undertake?
17 Are you forgetful?
18 Do other people think you are lively?
19 Can you get ready to go out within half an hour after receiving an unexpected invitation?
20 Do you like to have other people around?
21 Do you enjoy gambling?

22   Are you able to accept changes in plans without feeling upset?
23   Do you prefer dogs to cats?
24   Will you exchange casual glances with strangers rather than avoiding eye contact?
25   Are you willing to try out new brands of cosmetics or toothpaste?
26   Do you enjoy playing games at parties?
27   Do you usually feel well?
28   Do you like to meet people?
29   Do you like practical jokes?
30   Are you inclined to enjoy the drinks tonight without worrying about tomorrow?
31   Would you prefer to play drums rather than a flute?
32   Do your friends accuse you of never relaxing?
33   Are you good in an emergency?
34   Do you lose your temper easily?
35   Are you always ready to look ahead even when you have real personal problems?

Count up your yes answers and compare the number with your no answers. If you have more yes than no answers, you are extroverted. If you have more no answers, you are introverted. The greater the difference between yes and no answers, the more you are extroverted or introverted.

Extroversion is a trait description, and means that you turn your interest and attention to things, people and events outside yourself. You prefer the passing show to the contemplative life, society to isolation. But if you turn your interest and attention upon yourself, you are introverted.

Now, ask yourself a further question: Do you like spicy food? Does your answer seem to fit your answers to the earlier questions? In theory at least, if your answers were yes, you should like spicy foods, but if your answers were no, you should tend to like food relatively unseasoned.

Extroversion and introversion are extremes on a personality scale invented by the Swiss psychiatrist, C. J. Jung. Like Freud, his one-time colleague in the psychoanalytic movement, Jung sometimes sought physical explanations for behaviour. He considered that extroverts are more excitable than introverts. Professor H.J. Eysenck, who teaches psychiatry in London, has reversed Jung's physiological hypothesis. Eysenck has pointed out that about half of our brain cells inhibit the sending of messages by other cells. Only the other half excite cells to signal (see Chapter 2). He believes that extroverts are those people in whom the inhibitory activity of nerve cells in their brains overbalances the excitatory cells. Introverts are those in whom excitatory activity overbalances inhibitory activity. Thus, if you like spicy foods, perhaps it is because the nerve cells in your brain that register taste sensations require more excitation to overcome the inhibitory activity of other nerve cells, according to Eysenck, the foundation of an extroverted personality.

Eysenck is, of course, using the word, 'excitable' in a different way from Jung, to refer to the behaviour of cells rather than to the behaviour of the whole organism. His studies, using tests analogous to Game 1.1, indicate that introverts are more likely to become neurotic than extroverts. On the other hand, the old idea that hysteria is associated with extroversion does not appear to be true. Introverts are more easily conditioned than extroverts, presumably because their nerve cells respond more quickly to stimuli. Introverts tend to be less vigilant than extroverts and show less tolerance for pain. Extroverts are slower at rote learning, but introverts are more easily distracted from learning tasks. However, Eysenck recognizes that there is no clear demarcation between the two traits. They tend to blend into each other. Each of us is more or less introverted, less or more extroverted. In Game 1.1, very few if any readers will have all yes answers or all no answers.

As with the other personality traits described in this chapter, extroversion-introversion is a continuum. People differ in an infinite series of stages between one extreme and the other. Sexuality, intelligence and emotionality are each a continuum. No scale of sexuality is commonly agreed, but several stereotypes exist and will be examined in part two of this chapter. Intelligence ranges from the IQ grade 'Imbecile' to genius. We will explore the concept of intelligence in Chapter 4. Similarly, some of us tend to respond with laughter or with tears to situations in which other people merely smile or shrug. Emotional differences are discussed in Chapter 9.

Character traits are elements in a whole personality and ultimately it is the whole person which interests us. Think about yourself, about your own personality. Do you consider yourself clever? Are you interested in sex? Do you wish for love, and is not your wish as much an aspect of your emotionality as it is an aspect of sexuality?

Now, compare your personality to that of someone you live with or know well – a parent, spouse, lover or friend. Select a person and in your mind evaluate his or her personality in comparison with yours.

Game 1.2: You may find it useful to make the comparison using a scoring grid which also makes it possible to add other people to the game. Score each person including yourself on a scale from 1 to 10. Let 1 mean that the trait does not apply at all and 10 that it is a very good description.

	PERSON You	1	2	3	4
Extroverted					
Introverted					
Intelligent					
Sexually active					
Emotionally active					
Talkative					
Natural leader					
Disruptive in a group					
Independent					
Loving					
Gullible					
Tolerant					
Spiritual					
Trustworthy					
Brave					

You may also add traits to the list if you think it omits something important to you. Add up the score you have given each person. You have a rough comparison between your own personality evaluation and your evaluation of the others. You may find it amusing to ask them to play this game themselves. Compare their results to yours.

What you are doing is expressing your own opinion, how you see yourself and how you see others. But the important thing is that you are making a comparison. The other person has intelligence, sexuality, emotionality and is extroverted or introverted in 'quantities' that probably differ from yours. In a similar way the other person is probably taller or shorter than you are. They are heavier or lighter, darker-skinned or paler, more or less good-looking. Height, weight, skin-colour, and especially a trait as subjective as good looks, are also continua. People range along each trait on a scale from, let us say, 1 to 10.

Not all traits are continua. What colour are your eyes? What colour are the eyes of the person with whom you compared yourself? Eyes, or more precisely the irises of eyes, display a number of colour shades but the possible variations are far from infinite. Basically, they are blue, brown or grey-green. Eye colour is not a continuously variable trait. In fact, eye colour is inherited. The colour of your eyes was predetermined by your parents' with some variability within rigid limits beyond any known means of human control. Eye colour is a discontinuous trait. So is your blood type and several other facets of your immune-defence system, such as the rhesus factor. These too are inherited discontinuous traits which apparently cannot be altered by environment, experience or social manipulation.

The enzymes in your gut that digest your food are inherited characteristics, as are many of the hidden processes essential to life. On the other hand, few if any of the traits that identify us as individuals derive exclusively from the chemical composition of our parents' genes. All the multitude of traits that make you you and me me are influenced by our environments to a greater or lesser degree. For example, the average height of all the soldiers in the United States Army during World War I was 5 feet $7\frac{1}{2}$ inches. In World War II, twenty-five years or one generation later, the average height of all United States soldiers was 5 feet $9\frac{1}{2}$ inches. In 1917, perhaps one-fifth of the soldiers in the United States Army were immigrants from poorer, less well-nourished, less hygienic populations. By 1941, better food and better hygiene had done their work, and the average soldier had outgrown his father by two inches. This is stark evidence of the effect of environment on a physical characteristic, in this case height.

Many people assert that personality is affected by physical attributes such as height, weight, skin colour and condition, but that the essential facets of personality are 'mental'. It is your mind that is really uniquely you, or so it often seems. Bodies are fat or thin, flabby or muscular and generally too subject to wear and tear. Your mind, whatever its limitations, is you.

This way of looking at yourself is common enough, but is it right? No, it is not! It is arrant nonsense. Mind exists in a body. One's self-image is enormously influenced by the state of one's body. Even more to the point, mind exists in a physical organ called the brain. The characteristics of the brain, what it is and how its parts function, are the subject of later chapters. Here I want only to point out a fundamental fact: your brain embodies your mind. I am not talking about your soul, nor do I wish to. If you have a soul, its location and nature are beyond our knowledge, yours and mine. But without a brain, you have no mind. Indeed, there is no you. That is why in modern medicine the physical definition of death focuses on the brain, not the heart. Your heart can be kept beating indefinitely. When your brain dies, *you* cease to be.

Like arms and legs, hearts and stomachs, brains develop in fetuses because the genes dictate that they should. How this miracle comes to pass, no one yet knows. In the fetus, a neural tube forms in the first week after fertilization. What is to become the head end of this tube thickens as more nerve cells form the primitive brain. Probably this process in the individual fetus mirrors the development of brains in the course of evolution.

The physical development of each brain is influenced by the environment of the mother. A mother whose diet has been inadequate during her pregnancy may produce an infant deformed in some way, if it survives at all. The child's heart may be defective, it may be unusually small or its brain may be adversely affected. Such a starved child may learn more slowly than the offspring of a properly fed mother, but as yet there is no clear correlation between diet and brain size and structure. The fact is that the fetus drains an inadequately fed mother of those nutrients required for its growth, perhaps even putting its mother in real peril. What is more, the brain draws more than its fair share of any restricted nutrient supply. No one knows for sure why this should be the case, but the survival of the fetus at the expense of the mother is presumably nature's way of assuring the perpetuation of the species. By analogy, perhaps the brain is of first importance to the emergence of an individual capable of survival. Nevertheless, there seems little doubt that the mother's diet, general health and mental outlook have an effect on the fetal brain.

Therefore, the physical embodiment of the mind – the brain – appears to be subject to the environment from the beginning. Just as minds or brains are responsive to events around them, personalities also consist of traits, one formative element in which is inherited according to the physical laws of biochemistry while the other element in each trait is moulded from experience.

The infinite variety of personality stems from this duality. Your eyes are blue or brown or grey, but you are neither completely introverted not wholly extroverted. Everyone resists either permanent socializing or total loneliness. Some are more gregarious, some more shy.

Eysenck said that extroversion-introversion is related to cellular excitability. He referred to a characteristic shared by nervous and by muscle tissue, both of which are susceptible to stimulation. This is an inborn characteristic. Changes in the chemical surroundings of nerve and muscle cells causes them to behave like tiny electrical conductors and to change their physical states. Muscle cells contract. Nerve cells, called neurons, conduct a signal. Both are excitable. There is little evidence, however, that normal excitability varies significantly from individual to individual. Even less has it been possible to correlate supposed differences in excitability to a personality trait called extroversion-introversion. Various attempts have been made to locate those parts of the brain which cause us to feel extroverted or introverted but with little success. Eysenck believes that the traits are mediated by structures called the thalamus and the reticular activating system, both of them in the oldest parts of the brain, the parts humans share with other animals. More recent evidence suggests that the quality of introversion specifically defined as sensitivity to punishment is regulated in other brain regions. This evidence is based on operations performed on the frontal cortex, to remove a brain tumour, for example. After such an operation, the patient may become more introverted, but it may be as well to ask whether anyone who undergoes brain surgery may not feel oppressed not to say chastened for a long time afterwards? There is little neurophysiological support for Eysenck's theories.

Nor is there any good evidence that introverted parents produce introverted children, or indeed that the opposite is the case. Like any other personality trait, extroversion-introversion is best looked upon as a mixture of inherited brain physiology and experience, but without much hard evidence to delineate either factor.

II

It is a curious fact that in hermaphrodites, and often in normal pre-pubescent children, the left side is female in form and the right is male. The left side is more rounded, covered by less body hair and is less heavily-muscled than the right.

In women, furthermore, the left hand, foot and breast are often slightly larger than the right. In men, the right hand, foot and testicle tend to be slightly larger. Does the left side respond to female hormones and the right to male hormones? Could there be some truth in the stereotypic descriptions of men as logical and verbally-oriented? It is, after all, the left side of the brain that is responsible for the right side of the body, and in most of us the left side also regulates language functions. The right half of the brain, moreover, not only controls the left (female) side of the body, but is thought to govern the perception of colour, musical sound, learned emotions and possibly – a hint at the extreme complexity of the brain – skill in mathematics! Of course we all operate with a whole brain, not half a brain, but these differences suggest that there may be a relationship between brain structures and sexuality.

The following two games require the participation of as many of your family and friends as you can enlist.

Game 1.3: Ask each person to run through the alphabet in his or her head as quickly as possible, and to count the letters containing the sound 'ee' without counting on the fingers. Including the letter E, the correct answer is 9. Count up the mistakes made by each person and keep a record of them. You should find that the men make significantly more errors than the women. If you use a stopwatch to time your subjects, you may find that the women are also faster, but this difference is less clear-cut.

Game 1.4: Ask your subjects to count up silently and as quickly as possible, without using fingers, the number of typed capital letters that have a curve in them. They must be typed letters because some people write a capital A and others, an $\mathcal{a}$. The correct answer is 11. This time, the men should have made fewer mistakes and taken less time to give you their answers.

Note that not every one of your friends acts according to the average expectation, but on the first of the two tests, in general women will do better than men, and on the second the reverse is true. How can we explain this difference? The straight answer is, I don't know. But we can speculate. Possibly the relative importance of the right side of the brain, with its aptitude for musical sound, gives women an edge when it comes to counting letters sounding like 'ee'. Conversely, the shape of a letter may be a quality judged first by the left hemisphere, giving men the edge in the second game.

On the other hand, it could also be argued that the sound of a letter is the way to recognize it in speech, and speech-recognition is a left-hemisphere function. Or if you think again about the shape of a letter, in type it is far less individualized than in handwriting. Any real judgement of difference between the sexes, therefore, ought to be reflected in the written shape, but statistically that is not the case. Such contradictions show that speculation may be a useful guide for further research, but it is not a substitute for facts.

Game 1.5: In this test of sexuality, you are to measure your own judgement rather than the behaviour of other people. This is a subjective test. The last two were objective. The difference is important because the results of subjective tests and judgements are notoriously hard to evaluate, whereas objective tests have measurable results which should be repeatable. Yet a subjective test may tell us something interesting about ourselves.

The question you are about to answer is: How androgynous are you? On a continuum from masculine to feminine, where do you stand? Below are sixty traits. Indicate on a scale of 1 to 7 how well each trait describes you. A 1 means that the trait is never true for you, a 7 means that it is always true.

1	self-reliant	5	cheerful
2	yielding	6	moody
3	helpful	7	independent
4	defend own beliefs	8	shy

9	conscientious	36	conceited
10	athletic	37	dominant
11	affectionate	38	soft-spoken
12	theatrical	39	likable
13	assertive	40	masculine
14	easily flattered	41	warm
15	happy	42	solemn
16	strong personality	43	willing to take a stand
17	loyal	44	tender
18	unpredictable	45	friendly
19	forceful	46	aggressive
20	feminine	47	gullible
21	reliable	48	inefficient
22	analytical	49	childlike
23	sympathetic	50	act as a leader
24	jealous	51	adaptable
25	leadership ability	52	individualistic
26	sensitive to others	53	do not use harsh language
27	truthful		
28	willing to take risks	54	unsystematic
29	understanding	55	competitive
30	secretive	56	love children
31	decisive	57	tactful
32	compassionate	58	ambitious
33	sincere	59	gentle
34	self-sufficient	60	conventional
35	eager to soothe hurt feelings		

(a) Add up your ratings for traits 2, 5, 8, 11, 14, 17, 20, 23, 26, 29, 32, 35, 38, 41, 44, 47, 49, 53, 56 and 59. Divide the sum by 20. This is your Femininity Score.

(b) Add up your ratings for traits 1, 4, 7, 10, 13, 16, 19, 22, 25, 28, 31, 34, 37, 40, 43, 46, 50, 52, 55 and 58. Divide the sum by 20. This is your Masculinity Score.

(c) Subtract your Masculinity Score from your Femininity Score and multiply the result by 2.322. (This number comes from complex statistical procedures which are not relevant to the game itself.) You may end up with a minus number.

Now, locate yourself on the following scale:

Feminine	Near feminine	Androgynous	Near masculine	Masculine
2.025	1	0	-1	-2.025

◄───►

Of course, many people would hold that trait 1, self-reliant, is at least as much a feminine as a masculine trait. Because many of the qualities are subject to stereotypic bias, the test results may be subject to doubt.

Game 1.6: Here is another way of arriving at the same self-judgement of your sexuality. Imagine that you are leaving a restaurant. Just before you are about to open the door, a person of about your age taps you on the shoulder and says: 'Excuse me, but I think you forgot this umbrella.' What do you say? Will what you say differ depending on the sex of the person who stopped you? If the answer is 'yes', what does that tell you about yourself? Are you behaving in a manner that seems to you masculine, feminine, sexist, homosexual? Note that what you say in reply to the statement has nothing to do with whether the umbrella is yours, nor are the words themselves as important as whether you would have changed them according to the sex of the imagined person.

Subjective tests are fun and, as in Game 1.5, it is possible to build in a degree of randomization; that is, you are unlikely to remember the score you gave yourself for 19, forceful, when you get to 46, aggressive. On the other hand, practised games players will remember such little tricks and give themselves the same rating for both traits. Thus, subjective tests reflect your opinion of yourself, but very little about what others think of you.

Game 1.7: Here is another objective test that gives somewhat harder evidence. Ask your teen-aged friends of both sexes what percentage of their same-sex peers have had sexual intercourse. (You are asking for a percentage or a proportion, not who!) List their answers and take an average of the girls' and the boys'.

In one such test, teen-aged girls guessed about 66 percent of other girls had had sexual intercourse. Teen-aged boys said, about 91 percent! The actual figures in the groups questioned were 20 percent of the girls and 45 percent of the boys.

Teen-aged people appear to overestimate the sexual experience of their peers. What does that tell us about sexuality? Perhaps it tells us nothing that common sense has not already revealed; that is, that interest is seldom matched by opportunity. In other words, the objectivity of a test is no guarantee of scientific value. The question being asked must be relevant to the hypothesis being tested. Game 1.7 was supposed to test the hypothesis that your unique sexuality is part of a continuum – the hypothesis underlying this chapter. It fails to do this, but it may have some value as a demonstration that sexual judgements are coloured by desire.

Game 1.8: From the standpoint of their usefulness, subjective tests of personality can sometimes be more scientific than objective tests. For example, rank each of the following thirty personality traits with either an M, for masculine, or an F, for feminine. Go through the list a second time and check those traits which you think are desirable. You are making a judgement about the traits, not about yourself.

1	aggressive	11	logical	21	brusque
2	independent	12	worldly	22	gentle
3	emotional	13	businesslike	23	taciturn
4	objective	14	adventurous	24	sensitive
5	submissive	15	decisive	25	artistic
6	excitable	16	self-confident	26	sloppy
7	active	17	ambitious	27	quiet
8	passive	18	dependent	28	loud
9	dominant	19	conceited	29	secure
10	competitive	20	talkative	30	tender

Now compare your ratings with the following:

1	M	6	F	11	M	16	M	21	M	26	M
2	M	7	M	12	M	17	M	22	F	27	F
3	F	8	F	13	M	18	F	23	M	28	M
4	M	9	M	14	M	19	F	24	F	29	M
5	F	10	F	15	M	20	F	25	F	30	F

The masculine-feminine ratings against which you have compared your own are stereotypes based on ratings by a large number of men and women in the United States. What is more, the masculine traits were always considered to be more desirable, by and large, than the feminine traits. How closely do your ratings fit the stereotypes?

Against the stereotypes, consider the fact that in a traditionally male-dominated field, sport, in the twenty years between 1956 and 1976, Olympic records held by men fell very slightly. On the other hand, records held by women fell much more significantly. For example, the time for the men's 800 metres race fell exactly two seconds from 1.45:47 to 1.43:47. The time for the women's 800 metres fell from 2.05:0 to 1.54:94 – a fall of almost 10 seconds. Although no record in a women's event has been faster than the time in a comparable men's event, the women's speed record has come closer to the men's. Women began to run the 800 metres regularly in the Olympics only in 1960. Naturally, since then women runners have prepared for the event. In other words training has cut down the difference in speeds achieved by men and women. Training may never completely overcome physical differences such as musculature and fat distribution and men may always run a little faster than women, but the stereotypic conception of a slow, sinuous female gait has long since demanded modification. In fact personality stereotypes based on sexuality give little guidance to understanding real people.

Biochemical evidence supports the view that sexuality is a continuum. Everyone knows that hormones play a role in sexuality though no one knows exactly how they work. Women secrete the male hormone, testosterone, and men synthesize the female hormones, estrogen and progesterone. These three chemicals are structurally very much alike. The balance between them is different in the two sexes and helps to maintain the respective sexual characteristics. It is striking, however, that an injection of testosterone increases aggressive behaviour in both sexes. Progestin, a chemical like progesterone, causes the human male to become more passive, as one might expect, but it increases aggression in the female. Thus, aggression does not seem to be only the prerogative of the male hormone. Some preconditions must exist before progestin can cause aggressive behaviour. These preconditions may be due in part to experience. Perhaps this is the reason why the output of testosterone in the human male coincides with the period of ovulation in the menstrual cycle of the woman he lives with. There is also a correlation between the moods of cohabiting partners over a period of weeks, but this is perhaps not surprising. On the other hand, no relationship between fluctuations in mood and hormonal cycles has been demonstrated, with the possible exception of the symptoms often grouped together as pre-menstrual tension. At least as much evidence supports the argument that mood reflects environmental factors.

The brain centres directly affecting sexual behaviour are in a part of the old mid-brain called the hypothalamus. In animals, stimulation of the correct areas by means of microelectrodes implanted in the brain causes females to become receptive and males to ejaculate. There is also medical evidence that damage to analogous brain centres in human patients impairs their sexual behaviour.

Yet it is unwise to jump to conclusions. Though there are brain centres that appear to regulate sexual activity, knowledge about their functions is still too limited. In neurobiology there is a sin called reductionism; that is, the assignment of a behavioural function to a group of neurons. Wherever possible in this book, I will cautiously commit this sin by referring a kind of behaviour to a part of the brain. You must be skeptical. Sexual behaviour is a good case in point. True, without the relevant groups of neurons in the hypothalamus, a man can become impotent, but sexuality is a different trait from sexual behaviour as such. Whom you love, how often you have sex, what you do and how you feel are part of your personality. Your answers to questions about sexuality are probably almost entirely learned. That would help to make your peculiar combination of sexual traits unique.

III

Personality research can be a little like fortune telling. You say to the subject: 'You have a tendency to worry at times, but not to excess. True or false?' or 'Rate yourself on a scale from 1 to 7.' Most of us would probably accept the first statement as a description of ourselves. Similarly, when the fortune teller predicts that you will soon meet a dark stranger, you would have to live on a pretty deserted island to avoid fulfilling the prediction. Meeting a dark stranger is a remarkably common event. Of course, the fortune teller adds to the prediction a crystal ball, a darkened room, an odd costume and perhaps an accent, plus other accoutrements of magic and mystery. Well, science, especially psychology, does the same thing even if there is usually no intention to mystify. If someone in a white laboratory coat asks for your help, you feel pretty churlish and unsociable if you refuse to do what you are asked to do. So you look at the statement about worry and after some thought, you say, 'True'. In any other context you might have noted that 'You have a tendency to worry at times but not to excess' is almost meaningless as a trait description. What is a tendency? What is worry? How often is at times? What is excessive worry? No wonder an American psychologist, P. E. Meehl, has called the 'True' response a 'Barnum effect'. P. T. Barnum was the great American showman whose best known contribution to human wisdom was, 'There's a fool born every minute!'

Nowhere, I think, has the Barnum effect been seen to

better advantage than in the now famous experiments run by Stanley Milgram at Yale University as long ago as 1963. Milgram was interested in response to authority. For example, why did the Germans condone the murder of millions of their fellow citizens by the Nazis? How could the inquisitors, even with the backing of the British, get away with burning Joan of Arc? Why did American soldiers kill hundreds of Vietnamese women and children with flame throwers? (This actually happened after Milgram began his experiments, but it did happen.)

Milgram set up an experimental situation in which the subject placed himself under the direction of scientific authority. He was asked to help to find the limits of the pain people can endure, a meaningless question as we shall see in Chapter 7. The subject was told that he was to apply electric shocks of increasing strength to a second volunteer until the experimenter told him to stop. Subject one could not see the person receiving the shock, but he could hear clearly. The two subjects were introduced before the experiment began so that there had been personal contact, but they did not meet again in the laboratory. Subject one was told to increase the shock by turning a rheostat. As he did so, subject two began to tap his fingers and to move about. Eventually he moaned and cried out when the shock was administered. If subject one hesitated, the experimenter insisted that he carry on. The subject had agreed to the terms of the experiment, the experimenter said, and besides, the second subject was really perfectly all right. But the sounds of agony increased until either the experimenter called a halt or subject one refused to go on. Surprisingly few refused. The majority – both men and women – argued, protested, sweated, but did as they were told. Thus, the Barnum effect. The experimenter represents authority. Having accepted authority, the majority do as authority bids, no matter how barbaric. Subject one did not know that subject two was part of the experimental team and that no shocks were being administered.

But is there not perhaps a second Barnum effect hidden

within the first, one that Milgram had not planned for and failed to notice? He and many others have seen his results as proof that humans will abdicate their responsibilities for making a choice to any plausible authority. Yet many of the subjects, I think, responded not to a physical authority, the experimenter, but to an abstract authority, Science, the supreme authority of our late-twentieth-century world. They saw the value of scientific experiments as higher even than the sanctity of the individual. Unfortunately, naive people misunderstand the activities of science, especially the use of animals in painful experiments. Many of Milgram's real subjects seemed to extrapolate the idea of experimental pain to their own test situation. They said to themselves, in effect, if the importance of science warrants giving pain to animals then perhaps it is justified to hurt humans too. Either they forgot or they did not know that scientific ethics (and in England, the law) flatly forbid inflicting pain on animals, let alone humans. Had Milgram allowed subject two to experience an actual electric shock, he could have been sent to prison. It may have been because they misunderstood the role of experiment in science and not because they accepted authority that Milgram's subjects continued to inflict 'pain'. If that is so, Milgram was himself fooled by his results because he asked the wrong question. He asked whether subjects would always respond to authority. He failed to ask what authority they responded to, and for that reason, he did not ask whether they responded to myth or reality. I suspect that most of us accept that there is something greater than ourselves to which we owe respect if not allegiance: God or science. If that something is endangered, we may be brought to defend it. A human being may be the only animal which kills his own species without direct need or provocation, but humans are also the only animals with language and its related power to symbolize (see Chapter 6).

Three morals emerge from this cautionary tale. First, experimenters should be very careful to ask the right questions. Otherwise they may get the wrong answers.

Secondly, I think the acceptance of some authority beyond oneself is almost universal. Thirdly, and finally, we return to the understanding of personality. The degree to which we each need authority and the manner in which we each use the power authority invests in us varies infinitely.

This relationship to authority goes by different names. Adjustment and sense of security are two of the more common. One's degree of adjustment is expressed in everything one does. It is exemplified in our emotions and in how we get on with people, a process often called interpersonal relationships.

Game 1.9: Here is a list of personality styles and the message each of them is intended to convey to others. Which one suits you best?

Style	*Message*
The star (super-competent)	'I'm the best. Please applaud.'
The niggler	'Right or wrong, I know you're wrong.'
The victim	'Things never go right for me.'
The getter	'What have you got for me?'
The giver	'Hold still while I force-feed you.'
The driver	'Watch my smoke.'
The proud one	'I won't stoop to your level.'
The lion	'I am the king of the jungle.'
The mouse	'Don't frighten me.'
The martyr	'Look how I sacrifice for you.'
The critic	'You'll never make it.'
The unlovable one	'I'm not lovable.'
The undeserving one	'I don't deserve it.'
The person who wants to be above reproach	'Don't ever disapprove of me.'
The busy beaver	'If I don't do it, it won't get done.'
The baby	'I expect you to take care of me.'

The prince (princess)	'I'm special.'
The good person	'Be pleased by me.'
The computer	'These are the facts.'
The complainer	'Nobody knows the trouble I've seen.'
The tower of strength	'If I let up, everybody will fall apart.'
The hermit	'I don't need people.'
The excitement seeker	'Whoopee.'

The styles and messages are taken from a recent American textbook on personality. Do they not reveal an underlying cynicism which would make it embarrassing to categorize Christ Himself? Why should the authors have carefully avoided any positive styles or messages? If none of them suits you, can you describe your own style and what it says to the people around you?

Game 1.10: The following list of personality traits is based on a test series which originated in California. The traits are called Q items meaning Quotient, as in Intelligence Quotient (on IQ, see Chapter 4). The left-hand list defines positive adjustment, and the right-hand list defines negative adjustment. Construct your own adjustment profile by selecting the Q items – positive or negative – most applicable to you.

Positive

Has warmth, has the capacity for close relationships; compassionate

Is a genuinely dependable and responsible person.

Has insight into own motives and behaviour

Is productive; gets things done

Negative

Has a brittle ego-defence system, has a small reserve of integration; would be disorganized and maladaptive when under stress or trauma.

Feels cheated and victimized by life; self-pitying

Handles anxieties and conflicts by, in effect, refusing

Is socially perceptive of a wide range of interpersonal cues

Behaves in an ethically consistent manner; is consistent with own personal standards

Values independence and autonomy

Appears straightforward, candid in dealings with others

Able to see the heart of important problems

Genuinely values intellectual and cognitive matters

Calm, relaxed in manner

to recognize their presence; repressive or dissociative tendencies

Feels lack of personal meaning in life

Is self defeating

Vulnerable to real or fancied threat, generally fearful

Keeps people at a distance; avoids close interpersonal relationships

Basically anxious

Guileful and deceitful, manipulative, opportunistic

Subtly negativistic; tends to undermine and obstruct or sabotage

Behaves in a sympathetic or considerate manner

Has a wide range of interests

Hostility towards others

Tends to project his own feelings and motives on to others

Emotionally bland; flattened affect

Now for sense of security: as noted above, sense of security is another name for relationship to authority.

Game 1.11: This is a test of your adjustment which equates that trait with your sense of security. Two American psychologists, N. S. Enders and M. A. Okada, imagined four situations:

1   You are involved in dealing with other people whom you do not know well.

2   You may encounter physical danger.
3   You are in a new or strange situation.
4   You are involved in routine tasks.

For each of these four situations, rate yourself on a five-point scale from very much (1) to not at all (5) for the following 9 general statements, a total of 36 ratings (9 × 4).

1   I seek experiences like this.
2   I am perspiring.
3   I have an uneasy feeling.
4   I feel exhilarated and thrilled.
5   I have a fluttering feeling in my stomach.
6   I feel tense.
7   I enjoy a situation like this.
8   My heart beats faster.
9   I feel anxious.

Add up your scores for numbers 2, 3, 5, 6 and 9 for all four situations (20 scores; maximum possible score 100). Now, add up your scores for 1, 4, 7 and 8 (16 scores: maximum possible score 80). Subtract the second score from the first, and you have your own 'anxiety' score. If it is 1 or above (it can be as high as 20), you are insecure in that degree. If it is 0 or a minus number, you have a relatively strong sense of security.

With tests like Games 1.9 to 1.11, many psychologists have tried to construct a general theory of personality. They hope that such a theory will make it possible to predict behaviour. One recent textbook lists seven postulates which a theory of behaviour must encompass.

1   Behaviour is adaptive.
2   Personality is a learned pattern of behaviour.
3   Culture influences the patterning of behaviour.
4   Each person is unique.
5   One's personality determines one's selection of a response.
6   Understanding this pattern of selection permits prediction of behaviour.

7   Basic behaviour patterns permit an understanding of the
    specialized functions of behaviour, e.g., learning to drive
    or falling in love.

It is easy to criticize these postulates. For example, 2 and
3 are pretty much the same. Numbers 6 and 7 are not so
much postulates as theories. Yet the attempt to predict
behaviour is neither a waste of time nor necessarily only
the machination of a politician or an advertising account
executive. A satisfactory theory of personality might lead to
improved educational techniques. It might help to reduce the
incidence of mental disorders, particularly those which are
social in origin (see Afterword).

I doubt very much, however, that it is possible to have
a theory of personality, still less to predict behaviour,
until we know a great deal more about the human
brain. Note that the list of postulates omits any reference
to one's genetic inheritance though genes also influence
behaviour. Therein lies the real weakness of this list of
postulates. Any theory of personality must be anchored in
the body, especially the physical embodiment of selfhood,
the brain.

2 The Machinery

I

Short of do-it-yourself brain surgery, there is no easy way to experiment with the living brain. Its functions, in so far as they can be tested through behaviour, will be described in the later chapters of this book. Though you will have to do without games for the present (for exceptions, see pages 37 and 43), I urge you not to skip this chapter. The soup may be a little thicker, but it is all the more nourishing.

The human brain weighs about three pounds or 1300 grams. It represents about 3 percent of an average adult male's body weight. The female brain is a little smaller on average, but beware of drawing sexist conclusions. The dolphin brain weighs more than the human brain, both absolutely and as a proportion of body weight, but the dolphin cannot talk and lacks the behavioural repertoire of humans.

Despite its relatively small weight, the human brain receives at any one time about one-fifth of the blood pumped by the heart. It uses roughly the same proportion of the oxygen and nutrients carried by the blood. Indeed, the infant's brain may take as much as half of all the blood sugar, the principal source of energy for growth and normal activity. The brain's voracious fuel consumption is a measure of its importance in the body's overall regulation.

Yet unlike the heart, for example, the living brain looks absolutely still. Its highly convoluted surface is a shiny grey with pink lines showing the blood vessels. If the three-layered membrane containing the brain is punctured, the greyish substance flows out in a formless, viscous jelly. No interior membranes confine or define the brain's parts, but there are four cavities, called ventricles, in the centre of the brain mass. The ventricles are connected and lead into the cavity surrounding the spinal cord. The ventricle linings synthesize cerebro-spinal fluid (often designated CSF) which has several functions: it helps to diffuse nutrients, carries various essential chemicals and helps to cushion the brain and spinal cord against blows which shake the skull and body. The brain is suspended in the CSF, connected to the rest of the body only by blood vessels and great nerve trunks visible to the naked eye as thin, smooth white threads. The largest of these visible nerve tracts is the spinal cord. The floating isolation of the brain reflects its fragility. One of the commonest causes of accidental death is a blow to the skull which causes a build up of fluid pressure at the narrow opening where the brain stem leaves the skull to become the spinal cord. The pressure damages centres in the brain stem that regulate breathing and heart beat.

Brain tissue is by no means exclusively nervous tissue. About 80 percent of its substance consists of glial cells which support neurons and help them to function. Some glial cells synthesize a white, fatty material, myelin, which encases the long processes of many neurons, including those that connect the brain to the rest of the body. Myelin sheaths form the white matter in the brain and spinal cord. Glial cells probably also perform other functions, though these are not yet fully understood.

Of course, the neurons are the principal functional elements. In the mature human brain, there are some 10,000,000,000 or 10^9 neurons. New neurons are probably formed during the first year of life but not thereafter. Within limits, they can repair damage, but neurons do not divide like other cells and cannot replace themselves. After the age of about 20, some 10,000 neurons die each day so that brain weight declines with age to about 1000 grams at 70 years. The effects of this shrinkage on behaviour, and especially on memory, vary greatly from person to person.

Any one neuron can link up with as many as 250,000 others, and the average is about 60,000 connections. This enormous interconnectivity explains the complexity of the brain and the great difficulties facing research into the behavioural role of a part of the brain to say nothing of individual neurons.

II

One function of the neuron – its excitability – determines life as we know it. Every neuron consists of three parts, a little like the roots, trunk and branches of a tree (see Figure 2.1). The dendrites are the branches, dividing

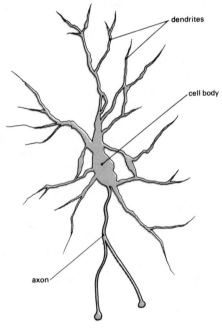

Fig. 2.1

frequently, thinning towards their tips and reaching out to make contact, or to synapse, with other neurons. Here the tree analogy breaks down, however, because the dendrites synapse with axons, the root-like processes of other neurons, and with their trunk-like cell bodies. The cell body contains the synthetic machinery forming the chemicals needed to make the neuron function. Out of the cell body, another process emerges called an axon. The axon may branch occasionally, but it does so far less often than the dendrites, and even the branches tend to retain their original thickness along their entire length. At its very tip, the axon swells slightly to form a bulb. All neurons consist of dendrites, a cell body and an axon, but the shapes they take vary enormously.

A nerve excitation, impulse or signal, originates at the place where the axon leaves the cell body. The excitation is sparked off because the dendrites and the cell body receive signals from other neurons. Sensory neurons at the periphery of the body, in the skin, for example, signal when the correct stimulus impinges on their specially-adapted dendrites. The signal consists of a flow of charged

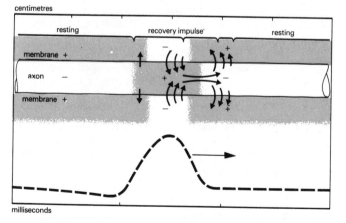

Fig. 2.2: The flow of ions into and around the neuron

atoms called ions. At rest, the inside of the axon is electri-
cally-negative with respect to the body fluid outside the
axon. When a signal begins, the membrane surrounding the
axon where it leaves the cell body changes its physical
properties. What happens exactly is not clear, but the result
is a flow into the axon of positively-charged sodium ions.
At about the same time, positively-charged potassium
ions begin to flow out of the axon but much more
slowly. The larger sodium influx causes the inside of the
axon to become neutral with respect to the outside, and
then because sodium ions continue to flow in, even more
positively-charged than the outside. This excess of sodium
ions inside the axon diffuses away from the cell body
causing the same membrane changes to occur sequentially
along the length of the axon, thus moving the signal
away from the cell body (see Figure 2.2). Meanwhile, the
outflow of potassium has stopped, and a further change in
the axon membrane causes sodium ions to be pumped out
again. Some potassium re-enters the axon, but after a brief
period during which the neuron is out of action, the
negatively-charged interior condition is restored, and the
neuron can send a second signal. Because the process
involves a change in electrical potential, in a manner
analogous to an electric battery, the signal itself is called an
action potential.

The action potential lasts from four to six milliseconds.
It moves along the axon at different rates of speed depending
on the thickness of the axon and whether it has a myelin
sheath. The sheath acts like an insulator. It is interrupted
at intervals (called nodes of Ranvier after the French
neuroanatomist who first described them) so that the action
potential does not flow along the axon but must jump from
node to node. In the larger, myelinated neurons, the signal
moves at about 200 feet per second, and in the smallest,
unmyelinated axons, at about two feet per second. In other
words, nerve signals are not instantaneous. Although they
can move from head to toe along at least four linked neurons
in a fraction of a second, there is a time lapse.

The nature of the action potential lays down several other conditions that are important for our understanding of how nerve signals move around in the brain. I have already noted the recalcitrant period during which the nerve cell cannot signal again. It lasts no more than three or four milliseconds, but it does impose an upper limit on the frequency of signals. It also means that each action potential must be a discrete physical event with a beginning and an end. During the action potential, the neuron is 'on'; between action potentials, it is 'off'. There is no in-between state (except that like most scientific generalizations, this one is not absolutely true; neurons may be more or less ready to signal, but the ultimate effect is still 'on' or 'off').

Every neuron sends exactly the same signal, an action potential. The question is, how do we tell one from another? How do we tell the difference between a strong light and a dim light, or between any light and a sound? There are three answers – and one large question mark, of which more below.

1 The more intense a stimulus – for example, the brighter the light – the more neurons send signals, and
2 the more frequently each of them signals.
3 Light and sound excite different neuronal pathways, those beginning in the eyes and ears, respectively.

Game 2.1: Close one eye. Use your finger, *not* a pen or pencil, to press gently against one corner of the eyelid. A patch of light will appear, probably in what seems to be the opposite side of the eye.

Pressure on the eyeball is carried through the viscous fluid that fills the interior to the retina, and is interpreted as light. You may 'see' the pressure in the opposite corner because of the way the optic nerve divides when it enters the brain (see Chapter 8).

Similarly, neurons are organized in pathways throughout the body. There is a pathway to bring touch sensation to the brain, for example, and another to conduct movement orders to the hand. Within the brain, the spinal cord and other nerve junctions called ganglia (singular: ganglion), pathways cross and signals may become mixed. Thus, especially in the brain, complex signal patterns are constructed. Sensations and the record of recent movements are mixed with memories, emotions and intentions.

Therein lies the great question mark about the interpretation of action potentials. How can an electro-chemical event – the action potential – look red, feel sad or push a typewriter key? Certainly, the transition from signal to psyche is essential for survival and the ability is inherited in the nature of the wiring. No doubt we also learn to distinguish between sensations and feelings, but learning is stored in memory. We are only postponing the search for an answer. Perhaps it will turn out to have been obvious all the time.

We have been talking about the action potential in a single neuron, and about pathways. In order for a pathway to exist, a signal must be transmitted from one neuron to the next. The nature of this event is at least as important as the action potential in determining the behaviour of the nervous system. When it reaches the axon bulb, the electrochemical signal is perforce halted. The membrane changes which have propagated the action potential now produce a new effect. Stored in the axon bulb are small molecules of a chemical called a transmitter. A few of these transmitter molecules are released into the synaptic gap between the axon bulb and the next neuron. Exactly how the release takes place is not clear, but there is little doubt that the nervous message is carried across the synaptic gap by the chemical transmitter. On the next dendrite, or cell body, it becomes attached by a chemical bond to a receptor molecule. The chemical bonding leads to an electrochemical change similar to that which initiates the signal in the axon. In the dendrite or cell body, however, this change merely alerts the neuron in a manner which is not completely understood. It may not cause an action potential to arise in the axon. In many, perhaps most, cases transmitter must be released from more than one presynaptic neuron to produce a post-synaptic action potential.

The process is complicated by another intriguing fact. Some of the transmitters cause the post-synaptic neuron to resist the electrochemical change that precedes an action potential. The post-synaptic neuron is inhibited by what is therefore called an inhibitory transmitter. Neurons that release inhibitory transmitters are called inhibitory neurons. Those that release transmitters which tend to evoke an action potential are called excitatory neurons. A single neuron appears to release only one kind of transmitter, but there are probably about the same number of excitatory and inhibitory neurons in the brain.

The post-synaptic neuron must be able to add up the transmitter signals it receives and to subtract the inhibitory signals. Because the great majority of brain neurons participate in more than one pathway, and are both pre- and post-synaptic neurons making thousands of connections, each neuron is perforce a calculating machine. It performs arithmetic and probably algebraic functions, and we can reasonably assume that this astonishing behaviour plays some role in the conversion of an action potential to psychological awareness.

Once the transmitter signal has been recorded by the post-synaptic neuron, the remaining molecules of transmitter must be nullified. They are either inactivated by being broken up by enzymes, or the transmitter is reabsorbed by the axon bulb. The synapse is thus cleared for another signal.

Note that malfunctions can happen anywhere in this system. A membrane can fail to initiate or transmit an action potential. Transmitter may not be available, or it may be incorrectly synthesized and therefore ineffective. Receptors may fail. Transmitter may remain too long in the synaptic gap. Each of these failures can produce the symptom of a disease. Perhaps the real wonder is that the system works admirably most of the time.

III

In the evolution of the nervous system, ganglia developed alongside the primitive spinal cord to serve the many functions required in each segment of a worm, for example. At the animal's front end, organs evolved to regulate the direction of movement, forerunners of a nose, ears and eyes. To serve these organs, a larger ganglion developed at the front end because there was more work to be done there. It became a brain.

Everyone accepts that the human brain developed out of these primitive anterior ganglia. Anatomically the brain has three parts, corresponding to its evolutionary stages, and, not surprisingly, functions have tended to move into the new parts as they appeared. (Purists would point out, quite correctly, that the new parts evolved simultaneously with the functions which they performed better than the old parts.) Heart and lung actions are regulated in the human hind-brain, the earliest part. The primitive analogue of the hind-brain must once have noted sensations and directed movement. In the human brain, sensation and movement are ultimately the responsibility of the newest part, the large cortex. Between the hind-brain and the cortex lies the mid-brain. Many mid-brain functions may well have originated with it. For example, anger, fear and body temperature are all regulated by the hypothalamus, a segment of the mid-brain. On the other hand the olfactory bulb at the front of the mid-brain, responsible for smell, has grown into the human cortex.

Over the centuries the naming of parts of the brain fell to the lot of anatomists who had to work with dead tissue. Often, they could not even obtain human brains, because of laws such as that which governed dead human bodies in Britain until 1832, and were forced to restrict their research to animal brains. Obviously, they were unable to relate structure to function so they had to fall back on appearances. The three evolutionary parts of the brain, plus a fourth, the cerebellum, are anatomically

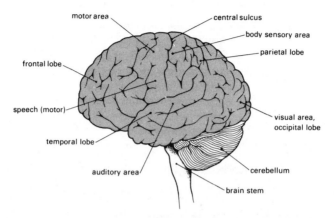

Fig. 2.3a: The human brain from the side

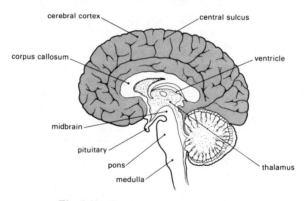

Fig. 2.3b: The human brain in section

distinctive, and the cortex is clearly split into two hemispheres (see Figures 2.3a and b). Otherwise the brain is undivided by bone, muscle or membrane. The naming of parts depends on grey segments defined by white matter and often further subdivided by shades of grey. Small wonder that the traditional brain parts seem to have little to do with function, but in the main the old names are all we have.

Broadly speaking, the old brain, composed of the hind- and mid-brain, regulates vegetative functions not usually under voluntary control. The new brain, principally the cortex, receives, stores and processes information and, with the cerebellum, regulates movement.

Cerebellum means little brain (see Figure 2.4). About the size of a child's fist, it is tucked beneath the occipital or rear lobes of the cortex on top of the hind-brain. Nervous signals reach it from the cortex via the mid- and hind-brain, and its nervous connections lead back through the hind-brain to the spinal cord. The cerebellum consists of regular arrays of a limited number of neuron types. All but one of these types are inhibitory. They modulate the signals that leave the cerebellum from the single excitatory type of neuron. Both its location and its structure suggest that the cerebellum mediates between the rest of the brain and the peripheral voluntary muscles.

It is the regulator of fine movement, especially learned movements such as playing the violin or driving a car. An analysis of the functions of cerebellar neuron types and the relationships between them has shown how fine movement control becomes habitual. It may be in part the cerebellum, for example, which permits a patient with damage to the language-control areas of the brain to write when he is un-

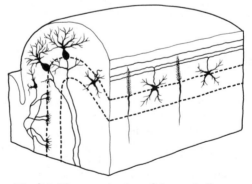

Fig. 2.4: The organization of the cerebellum

able to read or speak. This remarkable tissue has 'learned' to write. Damage to the cerebellum impairs or destroys movement sequences which cannot then be re-learned.

Cerebellar signals reach the spinal cord through the hind-brain. I have noted that the hind-brain regulates breathing and heartbeat, but these vital functions are also in part under local control. The heart has its own pacemaker and can operate independently of the brain. Lung function is also regulated by nerves that control the chest and diaphragm, including nerves under voluntary control which originate in the cortex. Indeed, there is evidence from yoga and the technique known as biofeedback that even heartbeat and brain waves can be brought under conscious control.

Game 2.2: Not everyone is able to play this game, but practice helps most people. Sit down and focus your attention on a picture, light source or sound, or a mandala if you are experienced at meditation. Your mind must restrict your attention to the selected object and the goal: either raising or lowering your heart rate. You will have to ask a friend to take your pulse at regular intervals. This action should be practised so that your friend becomes adept, and you become accustomed to the touch and can include it in your experience without disturbance. You and your friend should agree in advance how long each session is to continue, and the frequency at which he or she is to take your pulse. To avoid any later uncertainty, your friend should write down the pulse rate on each occasion. When the time is up for the session, your friend should gently attract your attention. You should both be aware that a few people can faint under the test conditions. Fainting is both infrequent and easily dealt with. Even if your position is awkward, providing it is not dangerous you should be left to lie as you are. Your friend should just loosen any restrictive clothing. Recovery comes rapidly.

On top of the hind-brain, tucked beneath the cerebellum, are four small lumps called colliculi (singular: colliculus).

Their functions are reminiscent of the original sensory-motor role of the old brain. The colliculi receive data through neurons connected to the eyes, ears and touch sensors throughout the body. The data from each sense arrive on neurons arranged in a map of the field, and the three sensory maps are juxtaposed. For example, your visual map designates things in your visual field at the moment – a tree here and a girl on the grass beneath it. About half the cells buried in the superior colliculi, the two upper lumps, receive signals from both the eyes and the ears. This ingenious arrangement provides an association area analogous to the human cortex for animals such as the frog, but what does it do for us? Perhaps it is an alerting mechanism. Suppose you are crossing a busy street. You are fully occupied with the oncoming traffic, unable to attend to the reverse flow on the other side of the road where a large lorry is approaching. The sound and sight of that approaching lorry will nevertheless impinge on your eyes and ears, signals will pass to the colliculi, and you will know that you must attend to an approaching object. The colliculi note something, but do not tell you what it is.

Running between the hind-brain and the mid-brain is a bundle of neurons called the reticular activiating system or reticular formation. This network consists of a mass of neurons connected directly to cell bodies as well as to dendrites by very short axons. Excitation spreads across the net in such a way that each neuron is affecting every other one. The all-or-nothing rule is effectively suspended, and the whole system modifies its state more slowly. Because of its location, its degree of excitation modulates the tone of the rest of the nervous system, the periphery as well as the brain. The physiological function of such a system can almost be guessed. When the reticular formation is excited, we are awake. When the tone is lowered, we sleep. If the reticular formation is destroyed, life continues but the patient is more or less deeply asleep.

In the mid-brain the first large structure connected to the reticular formation is the thalamus, a major relay point for touch and temperature data and for movement orders going out from the brain. The thalamus is connected to and modulated by a group of nerve centres called the basal ganglia (they are at the bottom of the mid-brain) with fine old names like putamen, caudate nucleus and substantia nigra (black substance, because it is darker than the surrounding tissue!). The basal ganglia regulate involuntary movements and help to sequence the operation of the hundreds of muscles which shape walking and facial expression. Damage to the basal ganglia or malfunction caused by disease underlie Parkinsonism and many other movement disorders.

Forward of the thalamus in the mid-brain lie two small areas of great interest. The amygdala and the hippocampus, with several smaller neuronal groups, form the limbic system. The amygdala is involved in emotional life. Damage to these cells may affect adversely our ability to control anger, fear or pleasure. Indeed, one of the latest surgical adaptations of the operation called a frontal lobotomy, for the relief of intractable depression, is destruction of a tiny area linking the limbic system to the frontal cortex. It is called a limbic leucotomy. Tranquillizing drugs which control mood are thought to work primarily in the limbic system. Recent reseach has discovered in this region of the brain a natural tranquillizer analogous to the natural opiate enkephalin. In other words, there may be a substance normally found in the limbic system which helps to prevent the abnormal agitation known as anxiety or depression (see Afterword).

Hippocampus means 'sea monster', and it was so named because an eighteenth-century English anatomist, named Phillips, fancied that the region looked like a sea horse. The hippocampus has been the subject of intensive study because it seems to play a role in learning, especially learning involving the space in which we live. It contains regular arrays of well-defined nerve cell bodies, and in animals action potentials can be accurately observed during a learning task by using tiny sensors called microelectrodes implanted near the cells. As part of the limbic system, moreover, the hippocampus is probably directly affected by mood in a manner which mirrors psychological experience of the relationship between mood and learning.

As its name indicates, the hypothalamus lies beneath the thalamus. No other bundle of neurons better exemplifies the folly of slavish adherence to the old names because the hypothalamus is a complex of several neuronal groups with related but diverse functions. Side by side there are centres regulating sensations of hunger and thirst and body temperature. Stimulation of nearby nuclei causes behaviour identifiable as anger, fear or pleasure. The pleasure may be so intense that experimental animals allowed to operate a self-stimulating apparatus via a microelectrode placed in their pleasure area will ignore food and water and continue stimulation until they literally drop from exhaustion. In view of its importance in the regulations of emotions, it is not surprising that the hypothalamus is linked to the amygdala.

Neurons in other hypothalamic centres produce hormones, chemicals which enter the blood and cause changes in tissues at some distance from the cells where they are produced. It is not clear whether these hypothalamic neurons signal in the normal way in addition to the added task that they have acquired. Their hormones act nearby on cells in the pituitary gland, and their importance can scarcely be exaggerated. Called releasing factors, the hypothalamic hormones cause the pituitary to release six or seven hormones of its own. They include ACTH (adrenocorticotropic hormone), which stimulates production of adrenaline, as well as hormones which regulate sexual activity, the menstrual cycle and growth. Thus, in addition to its role in the correlation of such fundamental drives as hunger and thirst with emotions, the hypothalamus helps to regulate basic body functions by means of non-nervous, chemical signals. Nervous signals are very fast and short-term whereas hormones act more slowly and over a long period. The hypothalamus provides the clearest evidence that mind and brain are inextricably intertwined.

III

If it were possible to flatten out all the ridges or gyri (singular: gyrus) and valleys or sulci (singular: sulcus) that give the human cortex its characteristically corruscated appearance, the sheet of tissue would be about the size of a normal pillow case. Its thickness varies, but on average it is roughly the same as that of a good bath towel. After the folds, its most obvious feature is its division into two halves or hemispheres. Many structures in the older parts of the brain are duplicated on each side of the midline, like the cortex, but the duplication is less obvious to the eye. The two cortical hemispheres are joined together by a great sheet of white matter called the corpus callosum. The split brains beloved of the media are actually brains in which the corpus callosum has been cut, dividing the hemispheres but leaving the mid- and hind-brain intact. Split brain surgery is performed on human patients only as a means of controlling severe epilepsy. It does so by isolating the hemisphere containing the epileptic focus so that the abnormal electric waves underlying epilepsy cannot spread to the other hemisphere. The study of the lateralization of functions, about which I have more to say below, has been advanced both by tests carried out voluntarily by these patients and by animal experiments, but it is important to remember that the normal brain is a single organ with a unified, interdependent cortex.

The cortex is further divided by six major sulci, three in each hemisphere, into eight lobes (see Figure 2.3a, p. 41). The occipital lobes at the back of the brain contain the primary visual centres to which light signals are conveyed. The parietal and temporal lobes are at the sides of each hemisphere, the parietal above and the temporal roughly below it. They are thought to process aural and visual sensory information, and on the forward margins of both lobes there are specialized sensory-motor centres. Their principal task is to initiate voluntary movement, but those in the temporal lobe may also play a role in involuntary

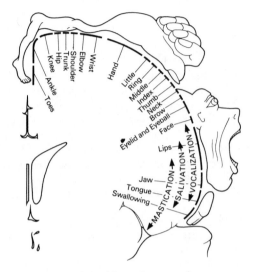

Fig. 2.5a: Motor homunculus

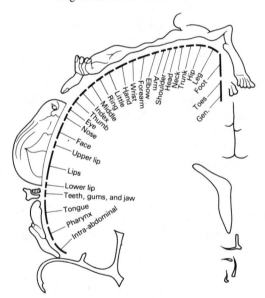

Fig. 2.5b: Sensory homunculus

muscular activity. The parietal and temporal lobes share the sensory-motor functions with the juxtaposed margins of the frontal lobes. Indeed, the primary motor areas are usually assigned to the rear margins of the frontal lobes and the sensory areas to the parieto-temporal, but the distinction is not so clear. Both regions probably perform both functions. What is clear, however, is the arrangement of the neurons which receive touch and temperature sensations, on the one hand, and those that direct movement on the other. Along each side of the sulcus – that is, on the rear margins of the frontal lobes and the forward margins of the parieto-temporal lobes – these neurons form a strangely distorted outline of the body called a homunculus (see Figures 2.5a and b). The feet are at the top and the head at the bottom. The hand area is enormous whereas the back area is quite small. The maps represent the number of neurons serving each area. Both sensation and muscular regulation are much more elaborate in the hands than they are in the back. This mapping, which we have already noticed in the colliculi on the hind-brain, appears also in the primary visual areas of the occipital lobes, where the maps represent the visual fields, and in other parts of the brain.

In the parieto-temporal lobes we find the clearest evidence of the phenomenon called lateralization. By and large, the right half of the brain receives sensory data from and regulates the activities of the left side of the body, and the left half of the brain, the right side. Except for the parieto-temporal lobes, both halves of the brain seem to perform the same functions for their respective sides of the body. In most people, however, the left parieto-temporal lobes regulate both the muscles involved in speech and writing and the ability to comprehend language, spoken as well as written. The right hemisphere in most people is adept at judging form, colour and non-verbal sounds, such as music. The lower right frontal lobe, moreover, appears to store learned emotions, for example, the pleasure or distaste aroused by certain smells. In some but not all left-handed people, the functions of the two hemispheres are reversed.

The earliest evidence of lateralization came from accidental brain damage. People who suffered wounds in the left side of their brains lost all or part of their language abilities. Damage on the right side, however, disrupted the ability to judge spatial relationships. But such losses are not absolute. If the damage occurs before the person is about fifteen years old, the impaired functions may be totally regained. As the human ability to learn implies, our brains are enormously plastic. Either they contain a large number of neurons which are not fully engaged, or within limits, neurons can change their functions. Even in adults, the loss of function due to brain damage may not be permanent. Some patients who have lost the ability to use language following left-hemisphere injuries, have been trained to proficiency in a sign language like that used by the deaf and dumb. It is thought that the sign language may call upon right-hemisphere skills.

Whatever the explanation for the recovery of language function, lateralization is still mysterious. Most of the data about it has come from the split-brain operations performed to treat epilepsy. After surgery, the patient shows neither intellectual nor gross behavioural deficits. However, if we suppose he is normally right-handed and cover his right eye, which is connected outside the corpus callosum to his left hemisphere, while showing him a spoon, he can describe the uses of the object but cannot name it. Give him the spoon to hold, so that touch sensations using pathways through the old brain to the cortex reach the left hemisphere, and he can instantly name the object. The patient knows what has been done to his brain. He knows in theory that if his right eye can see the object, he can then name it without touching it. Nevertheless, he cannot overcome the deficit until he can hold the spoon, or until the right eye is uncovered. Similar tests have revealed the form- and colour-sensing attributes peculiar to the right hemisphere.

To this limited degree, the patient may be said to have two brains. Can it also be argued that he has two

consciences? Only in the most abstract sense, I think, because even the split-brain patient thinks of himself as 'I',
never as 'we'. Perhaps it is more interesting to speculate
about the reasons why different data seem to be lodged in
different halves of a unified brain. Could there be different
kinds of neurons or some difference in the wiring of the
two hemispheres? Or could there be some difference in their
biochemistry? At present, we do not know.

Lateralization is only one of the unexplained mysteries of
cortical function. I have described so far regions that
account for roughly half of the cortex. In humans, all the
rest is the massive frontal lobes. Yet those functions which
have been localized – sensation, movement and language
– are to be found in the occipital, parietal and temporal
lobes and along a narrow band of the frontal lobes. Even
in the three rear lobes, large areas cannot be assigned
definite functions. These unassigned regions, the terra
incognita of the new brain, are usually called the association
cortex. In these regions, it is assumed that sensory data and
memory come together so that perception, thought and new
ideas emerge.

A Russian neuropsychologist, A. R. Luria, has described
one result of frontal-lobe damage in adults: the patient is
no longer able to direct his own behaviour. If he is
instructed, 'If you see a red light, press the button with
your right hand. If the light is green, press with your left
hand,' then whichever light first appears, the patient uses
the correct hand the first time, but will continue to press the
button with the same hand regardless of the colour of the
following lights. Similarly, if the patient is told to press a
button only when the red light is on, he begins to press
the button when the red light appears, but he does not
stop when it goes off or is replaced by the green
light. Luria wrote:

> these results mirror the results obtained with [normal]
> children ... of three or three and a half ... we were
> dealing with young people whose brains were still

developing. It is at this point that myelination of the neurons of the frontal lobe begins to reach completion; and it is at this age that young children begin to control their behaviour in accord with verbal instructions.

In other words, the damaged-frontal-lobe patients behave like children whose frontal lobes have not yet fully developed. Therefore, it appears that one function of the frontal lobes is to permit directed behaviour in response to language.

Perhaps there is a connection between this deficit following frontal-lobe damage and the well-publicized failure of the social senses in patients after frontal lobotomy. After all, the ability to obey moral and ethical precepts – that part of the mind which Freud called the Superego – is directed behaviour.

The first recorded evidence that the frontal lobes play such a role is the dramatic story of Phineas P. Gage. Gage was a twenty-five-year-old American foreman of a work gang building the Rutland and Burlington Railroad near Cavendish, Vermont, in 1848. They were using explosives to blast rock from the proposed line. The men had drilled into a large rock and poured powder into the hole. As was customary, Gage had the responsible and dangerous job of gently tamping the powder down before placing the fuse. A spark struck by the tamping iron ignited the powder. The explosion blew the three-and-a-half-foot long iron straight through Gage's head. It entered just below the left eye and emerged through the top of his skull landing fifty yards away.

Everyone assumed that would soon be the end of Gage, but he lingered on. Despite continuous bleeding, he recovered consciousness and said that night that he expected to return to work in a couple of days. Infection set in but Gage was up and about again in three weeks. Then it slowly emerged that the Gage who had survived the penetration of his forebrain by a massive iron bar was not the same man as the Gage who had placed the iron in that fateful hole. He was healthy enough and possessed all of his former strength but had none of the cheerful energy and sense of responsibility which had made him a popular foreman. He could no longer hold a regular job because added to his total undependability was a ferocious temper. For many years he lived by exhibiting himself and the tamping iron at fair grounds. Fortunately, when Gage died in San Francisco, his skull with its two great holes and the tamping iron were preserved. They are on display today in the Harvard Medical School.

That such gross damage should produce a gross disorder is hardly surprising. Still, it does not really help to understand the functions of the frontal lobes. In part, the problem is one of scale. In rat brains, about 85 percent of the cortex can be mapped and assigned functions. In human brains, about 85 percent has yet to be mapped. Fascinating attempts have been made. A Canadian brain surgeon, Wilder Penfield, performed experiments on normal unanesthetized patients which suggest that memory is a highly localized event. Because the brain has no sensory neurons registering pain, it is customary to perform brain surgery while the patient is fully conscious. A local anesthetic prevents pain when the skull is opened, and the patient is awake and able to answer the surgeon's questions, often an important guide in his delicate work. Penfield used a microelectrode to apply a mild electric current to the surface of the exposed cortex. His patients relived, in great detail, events which they could not recall consciously. When possible, the content of these memories was checked with people who were part of the event. Then, when Penfield's microelectrode was moved only a millimetre, the sensations would disappear and perhaps be replaced by others. If it was then reapplied to exactly the same spot, the same memory would reappear. The evidence seems to be very strong that each memory has an exact neuronal cubby hole.

Or does it? There is much more to be said about this fascinating puzzle in Chapter 5, but there is ample evidence that people have lost massive pieces of their brains without any observable loss of memory. An American psychologist, Karl Lashley, tried to resolve the problem by removing larger and larger segments of the brains of trained rats. He found that they suffered no loss of memory for the learned tasks until the damage began to impair their abilities to move. Professor Luria has written a fascinating book, *The Man with a Shattered World*, describing a patient whose memory was severely affected by a war wound which destroyed a large part of his left parieto-temporal region. Despite severe linguistic and physical impairment, the patient managed to keep a diary which Luria edited. The man had been a brilliant civil engineer. He had forgotten not just the details of his profession, but the faces of his family and the streets of his home town. He fought to write a journal in order to make himself a useful example to others faced with similar adversity. Thus, the patient had retained ethical and social memories despite the loss of the whole world centred around his language abilities. He also managed to write again, probably partly under the guidance of the automatic writing memory based in his cerebellum. Localization of memories remains one of the great uncertainties.

V

Because the neuronal signal is an electrochemical impulse, it is correct to say that the nervous system uses electricity. The idea that the electrical activity of the brain might be measured emerged at about the same time that its output of electrical energy was recognized. The electroencephalograph was developed in England during the 1920s. Today, the EEG is taken by attaching electrodes embedded in flat plastic discs to the top of the head and, usually, to the forehead and temples. Signals from each electrode are magnified and appear as a trace on a revolving paper drum or on an oscilloscope, an electronic tube similar to a television screen. The jagged lines of the EEG are hard to interpret, but specialists agree on the existence of four normal rhythms.

The alpha rhythm consists of slow, irregular waves and appears during waking periods of rest with closed eyes. When the eyes are opened and the attention focused, a short, rapid beta rhythm appears. Delta rhythms are long, regular waves associated with sleep. The deeper the sleep, the more pronounced the delta rhythm. The theta rhythm is unusual in adults, but occurs in children. It has also been observed during learning when microelectrodes have been implanted in the hippocampus of an experimental animal.

There is no mistaking the presence of these electrical signals. Some epileptics and patients suffering from certain other diseases display abnormal EEG patterns. The rhythms are helpful in distinguishing sleep states and in diagnosing a brain tumour. Yet the origins of EEG rhythms are not clear. Presumably, they reflect a summation of neuronal activity beneath the electrode, but no EEG component has yet been related to a specific group of neurons. On the other hand, the visual centres in the occipital lobes produce wave patterns in direct response to strobe lighting: the faster the strobe, the faster the wave, up to thirty per second. The EEG may reflect some combination of internal brain state and environmental influence.

And so it should. The brain is most notably the organ which correlates the environment to the body state, and vice versa. If you are hungry, the brain notifies you of the fact and organizes your journey to the kitchen and what you do there. If you are threatened, the brain draws on memory and other physical resources, such as muscle, for defence or escape. The French physiologist, Claude Bernard, said 150 years ago that living matter seeks to achieve a balance in its vital activities. For example, every organism must balance the output of energy with its intake. Fifty years ago an American physiologist, W. B. Cannon, called this process homeostasis. The homeostatic organ par excellence is the brain.

3 Consciousness

I

Game 3.1: When you are not thirsty, drink two glasses of water. You should soon have to urinate. If you collect the urine, you will find that about two full glasses are excreted within half an hour after you drank the water.

An adult has roughly 45 litres of fluid in his body, including blood, lymph and extra-cellular fluid. The addition of two glasses of water, about 500 ml, increases the amount of body fluid to 45.5 litres. Most of the addition goes into the blood. The result is an increase in osmotic pressure from the blood through the capillaries into the extra-cellular fluid. Osmo-receptors – neurons that sense osmotic pressure – in the hypothalamus reduce the synthesis of the hypothalamic hormone which causes the pituitary gland to produce anti-diuretic hormone (ADH). Diuresis is the process of fluid clearance, primarily through the kidneys. After you have drunk the 500 ml of water, less ADH is needed, and fluid excretion increases. The additional liquid has reduced production of two chemicals so that your body fluid volume can rapidly return to normal. This regulation is an excellent example of the feedback control operating through the brain to maintain homeostasis. The chemical-nervous loop is involuntary and unconscious, two sides of the same coin. Your feeling of thirst or satiety, on the other hand, is conscious, and it is evidence that consciousness like mind is merely a reflection of matter.

Consciousness is what the brain is all about. Homeostasis may be its weekday labour, but consciousness is the bonus bestowed by excess capacity. But how? I am I. What, then, am I, or rather, what is 'I'? This question gives much of the point to brain research. When the 'I' is disturbed by disease, medicine seeks a cure, first in the body (including the brain of course), and then in the ultimate product of the brain, consciousness. Even so, brain scientists are reluctant to deal with large, poorly-defined concepts. Although they will usually acknowledge that a description of consciousness is what they would ultimately like to achieve, they prefer to study movement, sensation, perception, even memory and learning, because these are more precise attributes.

Game 3.2: One of the better examples of the importance of self is called 'the cocktail-party effect'. You can try it the next time you are going to a crowded affair where there will be lots of noisy conversation. Ask a friend who is going to the same party to inject your name – your full name, if possible – into his conversation when he is out of your sight and at some distance from you. If possible, he should select a moment when you are chatting to someone else. He is to speak as quietly as possible providing only that he can be heard by the person he is addressing. If you do not respond the first time, he is to repeat your full name a little louder until you do hear him. He may have to explain to his companion what is going on, but there is every chance you will hear your name the first time your friend says it.

You will have known what is to happen, but the effect can be observed even without prior knowledge and is quite common. Your name, being very important to you, immediately attracts your conscious attention. In this sense consciousness is highly selective. You attend to whatever is relevant to yourself. Much of the chatter at the party was irrelevant as far as you were concerned. You heard it, but because you paid no attention to it it slipped quickly out of memory. In fact, it may never have reached memory at all.

By attending to them, normally unconscious activities, both of mind and body, may be illuminated. You can become aware because you have made the event important even though it usually goes on beneath the conscious level. According to Freud, verbal slips and similar accidents provide clues to the understanding of the self; they reflect an unconscious activity which can be made conscious by attending to it. If you know someone well, why should you suddenly forget her name? If you want to call one of the children, why do you name them all before naming the right one? Freud may have overstated his case, but by making the little mistakes important, he made us aware of them. The next time you mis-speak, ask yourself what the mistake was and why it happened? You may not get an answer, but if you do, it could surprise you.

Psychoanalysis was designed to draw out of the unconscious lost events, though it must be admitted that Freud said they were repressed not because they lacked relevance but rather the reverse. Still, if the lost event was painful, as Freud supposed, it could be repressed to protect the self. Freud's theory is not necessarily inconsistent with the modern view of consciousness, but Freud raised questions about pain and protection which carry us even further into speculation and uncertainty.

Reflex actions are physical examples of activities that can be brought into consciousness by focusing attention on them. The first reflex action to be described, by a Scotsman named Whytt in 1751, is called the pupillary reflex.

Game 3.3: You can observe the pupillary reflex without difficulty. Look at your eyes in a mirror in a dimly-lit room. Notice how large your pupils are. Continue to observe your eyes in the mirror and ask a friend to flood the room with as much light as possible with one switch. He might even shine a bright flashlight directly into your face. Your pupils will contract quickly.

Although a very bright light can feel painful, the pupillary reflex is not essentially protective. It increases visual acuity under the conditions of bright light. The smaller your pupil, the more the image is focused on to a limited number of the most highly sensitive receivers (see Chapter 8). In a dim light the larger pupil permits the image to spread across more receivers. Acuity declines accordingly, but your chance of noticing any movement in the field of vision improves.

The pupil itself is just a hole and does not change size. It is the iris, the coloured ring of muscle around the pupil, which contracts or enlarges. The reflex is produced by light signals to the colliculi on the hind-brain whence a signal is relayed directly back to the iris.

Unlike some other reflexes, the pupillary reflex cannot be brought under voluntary control. Yet it is affected by the degree of attention and by the emotions (see Chapter 9). When your interest is high, your pupils enlarge, a fact which clever traders exploit in dealing with a customer, and poker players also understand.

Game 3.4: You will need some pictures of nudes and a co-operative friend to whom the pictures will appeal. You should be seated comfortably opposite to one another in a good light so that you can watch your friend's eyes without being obvious about it. Your friend is not to know the object of the game beforehand. Now, pass one of the pictures to your friend and observe his/her pupils. They should grow very large at once. If they do not, you may have learned something new about your friend! (If your friend might be distressed by self-revelation, he/she should not play this game.)

The conditioned reflex is so-called because it is created or destroyed by conditioning, a form of learning (see Chapter 6). Once it exists, the reflex is no less automatic than any other reflex, and it probably arises out of some physical change in nervous connections. Because it is learned, however, awareness can modify its impact. These generalizations are well illustrated by an experiment conducted in America with six-month-old puppies. These demonstrations also make it pretty clear that consciousness is by no means exclusively a human attribute.

The puppies were starved for two days. Then they were placed in a room with the experimenter and two bowls, one filled with boiled horse meat and the other with a commercial dog food. Most of the puppies went at once for the horsemeat, but as soon as one touched it the experimenter swatted him with a rolled up newspaper. If one tap was not enough to make a puppy withdraw, more were administered until the animal gave up and ate the commercial food instead. This they were allowed to eat in peace. The training went on for several days until most of the puppies went directly to the commercial food as soon as they entered the room.

When the puppies had been conditioned to ignore their normal preference, the experimenter did not enter the room with them. The puppies found the two bowls but no minatory human being. As before, they ate the commercial food, but then their real travail began. The dish of horsemeat beckoned. According to the experimenter, an American psychologist named Solomon: 'Some puppies would circle the dish over and over again. Some puppies walked around the room with their eyes to the wall, not looking at the dish. Other puppies got down on their bellies and slowly crawled forward, barking and whining.' Solomon measured their ability to resist temptation in the time elapsed before one ate the forbidden food.

On the next day the puppies found only the bowl of horsemeat in the room. If any puppy did not eat from it within half an hour, the puppy was removed and not fed that day. The following day the puppies were again offered the horsemeat in the experiment room for half an hour, after which they were taken back to their cages. This continued until every puppy either broke the law by eating the horsemeat or, if one simply could not overcome the taboo, it had to be fed to be kept alive. The 'weakest' puppy ate the horsemeat in six minutes. It took the 'strongest' sixteen days!

Why this variability? What do I mean by equating 'strong' with law-abiding and 'weak' with law-breaking? Perhaps the two questions have the same answer. The puppies' natural inclination – their unconditioned reflex – was to gobble up the horsemeat. Conditioning turned this around and made the taboo a powerful and automatic response. Some puppies were much more easily conditioned than others. They tended to be 'strong' and to obey the law even at risk to their lives. Other puppies resisted conditioning. They tended to be the ones that broke the law as soon as the policeman was withdrawn.

According to the best available evidence, based in part on learning behaviour in octopuses, conditioned reflexes require the facilitation of neuronal signal transmission at certain synapses. That is, although the link between two neurons existed before training, some change in either or both neurons brought about by the training makes the link work more easily, like a valve that has been greased. When the conditioned reflex is extinguished – that is, when any puppy eats the horsemeat – it is supposed that the physical change in the synapse has either been reversed or, and this seems more likely, it has been inhibited by the new conditioning. The variability in the time required to bring about the physical change which wipes out the original conditioned reflex may depend in part on a genetic predisposition. In some puppies the synaptic change takes place more readily than in others, according to the theory. These puppies would be more easily conditioned and would find it hardest to unlearn the original lesson. They would be the last to break the law. The criminal puppies, on the other hand, develop conditioning more slowly and relearn more rapidly.

But beware. Not all learning is of the same nature. Being a quick study at one learning task is no guarantee that your neurons make you a genetic genius.

From the standpoint of consciousness, the important part of this story is the nervous machinery. Although different kinds of learning probably involve a variety of physio-chemical changes in neurons, synaptic facilitation underlies conditioning. Like the pupillary reflex, a conditioned reflex follows a well-marked neural pathway. The conditioned pathway may be much more complex, however, involving more neurons and more synapses with the far greater possibility of stimulating signals in pathways not directly involved in the reflex. Speculative though it is, you can imagine that a signal originating in a conditioned stimulus will not only produce the expected conditioned response, but will also reverberate through other circuits. Given the all or nothing response of each successive neuron, the signal may continue until it is stopped by inhibition, or because it is insufficient to stimulate further signalling. During the reverberatory period, one circuit could produce attention. Another might stimulate neurons in the language regions of the left parieto-temporal lobe, producing symbols. The symbols can express hunger or sexual arousal, both elements in consciousness. The symbols apply to or imply a 'Self'.

Incidentally, it is interesting that those of Solomon's puppies which had been hand-fed from the time they were weaned were the 'strongest', the slowest to break the law: their conditioning lasted longest. The conditioning of machine-fed puppies was extinguished much faster. Perhaps this is evidence for the relationship between handling and attention in early life and the smoother socialization of the individual. But the phenomenon raises a serious doubt about any fixed genetic characteristic of the neuronal synapse affecting conditioning. If early care is relevant, then the rapidity of the physical change at the synapse must be altered by experience. Nevertheless, consciousness would appear to be a consequence of the almost accidental multiplication of circuits, whether they are organized by inheritance or environment.

Finally, the good and bad puppies recall the personality trait described as extroversion-introversion in Chapter 1. Extroverts are said to condition poorly, and introverts more easily. Without trying to decide which puppies were extroverts and which introverts (although any dog owner knows that the terms are perfectly applicable), it is worth noting again that the ease with which they accepted conditioning was related to the way they were weaned. Extroversion-introversion is a continuum altered by environment, like any other trait, and the entire structure of the personality becomes involved when choices must be made.

Awareness and attention are matters of choice, and they occur within a context of purpose. A. R. Luria has pointed out that any action calls into play a system of behaviour which includes purpose as well as sensation and motion. Consciousness contains the ultimate awareness of one's goals. In some of the experiments by the American physiologist, Karl Lashley, it was found that even a rat with severe brain damage would get to where it was going despite the loss of normal walking, if necessary by rolling head over heels. Writing done with either hand or with either foot, for that matter, says what the writer wants to say and may even reveal characteristics of the writer's normal handwriting.

Game 3.5: Try writing with your foot. Compare the result with your normal handwriting. With practice, you should find that there are similarities in the way you form letters no matter which extremity you use.

When you drive a car, you shift gears automatically because you no longer need to attend to the action. Driving is highly goal-oriented behaviour in which you may be aware only of the object of the journey. Behaviour is never an indivisible response localized in one place in the brain. Unless the individual is seriously ill, his behaviour is always part of a goal-directed system. The whole system is often summed up as consciousness.

II

Implicit in the discussion of goals is an aspect of consciousness which we can call continuity. Each of us lives in a time dimension. We have a past and a future as well as a present. Our goals always exist in the future until they are attained.

Game 3.6: You can demonstrate the 'now-ness' of consciousness if you have a metronome or a loud clock or some other device for producing a regular series of sounds that can be varied and interrupted. How many beats are 'now'? The amount of now you can encompass depends on the speed of the metronome and the grouping of its clicks; that is, the presence of rhythm. The faster the clicks, the less you seem to be able to retain. But if a rhythm is imparted to the beats, like the rhythm you give to railway wheels when the train is moving, now becomes almost infinite. Time is forgotten. You hear the rhythm as a whole, like a whole song, until it is interrupted either by stopping the clicks or by some other interruption. This demonstration, by the way, is among the oldest in the field of psychology, having been introduced more than a century ago by the German, Gustav Theodor Fechner (see Chapter 7).

Perhaps the continuity of consciousness seems to you to be a fairly obvious quality. Whether or not we are the same people at sixty as we were at twenty, we always insist upon the existence of a unitary self. People around us agree, furthermore, for better or worse. It is possible, though, to clothe this somewhat abstract quality in everyday dress.

Game 3.7: Can you awaken yourself in the morning at a predetermined hour? With a little practice, you can, providing you have had a good night's sleep. Many people find that they need a bit of play-acting just before sleep. You may find it effective to draw on your forehead a clock showing the time you want to awaken, but use your finger rather than a pencil! Some people just write the number of the desired hour on their foreheads. Another trick is to bang your head against the pillow the appropriate number of times, for example seven times for 7:00, but half hours can be a problem. Or as you drift off to sleep, imagine a large clock and yourself dragging the hands around to the correct hour for awakening. At first you may miss by an uncomfortable margin, and you may wish to use an alarm clock as a standby, but very soon you will awaken right on schedule.

Now, it seems a reasonable argument that the trick of awakening at a predetermined hour would be impossible unless the self carried on through sleep. If this game seems to be a trivial way of getting at such a big point, then try to imagine what kind of nervous machinery counts the minutes for you during sleep. Although the skill of awakening yourself on time can be learned, it must be founded on an inborn capacity to measure duration. Biological clocks no doubt exist, as the menstrual cycle demonstrates, but the problem with awakening by using them is their multiplicity, and the fact that no two of them tell the same time (see Chapter 10). Part of the problem of what happens to consciousness during sleep is the nature of sleep itself.

Without sleep, people become irritable and inefficient. If sleep deprivation goes on, serious mental disorders develop. Like oxygen, food and water, sleep is a physical necessity. Yet the function of sleep remains a mystery.

Various theories exist. The late Christopher Evans, an English neurophysicist, suggested that sleep provides the breathing space needed by the brain to absorb the new data of the preceding day into the memory banks. In Evans' computer analogy, the brain goes off-line during sleep. Dreams reflect the reprogramming initiated by new experience. Unfortunately, there is very little evidence to support this rather pleasing hypothesis. It is, incidentally, directly opposed to Freud's explanation of dreams. He said that they are a sort of safety valve conducting energy away from the waking mind so that sleep becomes possible. In other words, you dream in order to be able to sleep. But Freud had no specific theory about sleep itself. Along with the rest of us, he seemed to accept that sleep 'knits up the ravelled sleeve of care', the common view that without sleep muscles cannot mend and the brain loses energy.

Within limits, the common view is true enough. For example, students who get a good night's sleep before an examination do better on average than those who have less sleep or none at all. Muscles certainly need rest to achieve peak efficiency, but there the common wisdom loses experimental support. Tired muscles recover peak efficiency almost as quickly with non-sleeping rest and relaxation such as putting your feet up. There is no unequivocal evidence that growth is slowed by sleep loss. Even the apparent relationship between sleep and mental efficiency is puzzling because the brain does not really sleep. The ability to awaken oneself at a predetermined time is evidence of this. The brain seems always to be aware of the world at some level. Indeed, it would be a most inefficient animal that laid itself completely open to attack for even a brief sleep period. (Hibernation is a different physical state and usually occurs in a well-protected shelter.) Sounds, touch, smells and even light become parts of dreams. There are few parents who do not awaken instantly to the cry of their child. In addition to this homely evidence that the brain never sleeps entirely, there is supporting physiological evidence. Its consumption of glucose and oxygen are the same or only very slightly lowered during sleep. These substances are the source of cell energy, suggesting that nerve cells must still be working. Though the EEG rhythm of sleep differs from waking patterns, it implies that cells are still signalling.

There is a good deal of evidence that neurons do not work at random, either, but that they operate in groups or perhaps along pathways such as those established during conditioning. This could provide a physiological explanation of dreaming because dreams are an ordering of events, however odd their sequence. Non-random nervous activity could also underlie the hallucinations that characterize the isolation of the body from normal sensation during sensory deprivation or in the delirium of illness. If it is true moreover, that schizophrenia reflects severely-disordered perception, the hallucinations associated with this disease may also be the manifestation of non-random nervous activity. Thus, the Freudian insight into dreams and sleep could have been profound: the continuity of consciousness is never really interrupted, but one's attention shifts from the Ego in waking to the Id in sleep and disease.

Game 3.8: The next time you awaken in the middle of the night, focus your attention on wakefulness. Keep your eyes closed and try not to touch anything except the bedclothes. Lie as quietly as you can and relax. If you do not drift off to sleep again immediately, you may notice that something is happening to you: some niggling worry from the day before will recur to you and grow larger and larger until you actively push it away from you. Or you may feel vaguely anxious and unhappy, an almost contentless depression. You can stop this too if need be, but you will probably just fall asleep again before the mood becomes too unpleasant. Such moments, usually very brief, are probably the effect of relative sensory deprivation. A 'you' occupies your body that is somehow unreal. No wonder more deaths take place between two and four in the morning than at any other time. Nor is it surprising that in many mental illnesses, sleep is severely disturbed, especially during the second half of the night.

The theory of non-random nervous activity may be useful, but it does not really take us very far towards understanding dreams. It is possible to dream at any time, but most dreams occur during a well-defined phase of sleep which recurs at roughly 90-minute intervals during the night. Far from being the mysterious dramas of Jungian myth, moreover, most dreams actually take place in the dreamer's home and deal more or less explicitly with events of the last day or two. A few are outlandish. An allegedly symbolic dream about incest may be followed on the very next night by a shockingly frank dream of the incestuous act. People starved for several days dream about food no more often than do those who have been eating normally. On the other hand, the eyes of a sleeper dreaming about climbing steps may flick upwards just as our eyes do when we climb steps during waking life. So what does determine dream content? More than eighty years after Freud wrote *The Meaning of Dreams*, we are no closer to an answer than he was.

Many people say they do not dream. The evidence suggests that they do, that everyone dreams. Dogs, cats and many other animals almost certainly dream too. People often forget their dreams, but with a little practice it is possible to prove to yourself that you do dream. Say to yourself before sleep that if you dream, you will awaken when the dream ends. If you also want to remember what you dreamed, then when you awaken – and you will – force yourself to turn on the light and write down the dream. After a few such efforts, you will find that even if you allow yourself to sleep through after a dream, more than one will come back to you in the morning. Now, you can begin to consider your dream content.

Game 3.9: This game works on the theory that consciousness is continuous, and that you are the best judge of your own goals. For purposes of interpretation, the sooner after a dream you wake up the better because more details will remain with you. First, try to note your feeling about the whole dream. Were you frightened, uneasy, sad, amused, pleased? Occasionally, you will awaken with no feeling at all about the dream. In any case, after grasping the feeling, recall as many details as you can: who was there, what happened, where, what things were present, what was said, and so on. For the moment, ignore the sequence while you try to collect the details. Then quickly, arrange them as closely as you can in the sequence of the dream. All of this should take about a minute and by the time you have finished, you should have the 'meaning'. Do not search for something mysterious or symbolic. Perhaps it is merely an event that took place the previous day, only in the dream you find that it made you anxious. Was it the feeling that you failed to notice when the event actually happened? Or you dream about your companion and awaken with a sense of pleasure. Yet you have gone to sleep after a violent argument. The dream meaning seems pretty clear. Or you dream the solution to a problem you have struggled to solve during the day. It does happen, perhaps because daytime distractions have been withdrawn. Occasionally, the dream will seem to contain a detail that you cannot explain or fit in. Leave it alone. It may yet fall into place, but if not, could it be that the detail has become misplaced from another dream? No one is sure that the non-random activities of neurons must make sense.

Nor does anyone know what non-random means in a physiological sense. Sleep is a state occurring when chemical changes in the reticular activating system slow down neuronal activity in the system. Perhaps because the body is immobilized, the sensory-motor centres are relatively free from stimulation. Association centres, including emotional centres, are also released from immediate use and therefore produce their own activities.

It is clear that sleep consists of at least four phases. Dreaming occurs regularly in only one, REM, or rapid-eye-movement sleep, so-called because the sleeper's eyeballs can be seen to move beneath the closed eyelids. During this sleep phase, the EEG contains a high proportion of the waking alpha rhythm. Breathing and heart rate are similar to waking, and erections occur. Although REM sleep looks like a preparation for awakening, three or four times during the night it is followed immediately by the deep sleep phases which then lead again to REM sleep. Only at the end of a normal sleep period does REM sleep lead into wakefulness.

On going to sleep the brain slips swiftly through phases two and three into the deepest sleep, marked by long, slow delta rhythms. The earlier deep sleep phases are distinguished only because the EEG has less delta rhythm. Breathing and heart rate are slow and shallow. Paradoxically, there is some evidence that sleep walking occurs only during deep sleep. Nervous transmission through the pyramidal tracts of the brain, tracts of neurons primarily concerned with regulation of involuntary movement, is slower in deep sleep than during waking. About four-fifths of the night is normally divided roughly equally between the three phases of deep sleep. After sleep deprivation, moreover, the catch-up effect is directly related not only to the gross number of sleep hours lost but also to the phases interrupted. Thus, barbiturate drugs can bring on and perpetuate sleep, but they significantly reduce REM sleep. When the drug is stopped, the subject experiences an unusually high percentage of REM sleep. Similarly, if deep sleep is interrupted, the later sleep periods will contain significantly more of the phase lost. Evidently, the sleep phases are balanced by a sensitive regulator, but what or where it is remains a mystery.

How much sleep is enough? Dogs and cats can manage with two or three hours a day, and rats and mice with less. Primates require more. Humans, with the most complex brains, require more sleep than any other species if you omit hibernation. Adults need roughly eight hours sleep in every twenty-four. Practice and necessity can produce variations, and there are people who seem to be well served by six or seven hours. But the Napoleon who sleeps four hours a night for weeks on end usually manages to take cat naps on horseback. There are differences in sleep needs, but they are less extreme than one is occasionally led to believe.

Infants do sleep much more, of course. Without better information about the reasons for sleep, it is not easy to say why. Their brains are growing inside their growing bodies, and because the newborn sensory apparatus is still growing, the infant lives partially shut off from the world. Infant temperature control is erratic, for example, and the apparatus of sight matures after birth. If this is a reason for infant sleep, it might also have some bearing on the longer sleep periods of the very old. Their sensory apparatus is increasingly inefficient. Perhaps the old are forced to spend more time within themselves too. In both the very young and the very old, consciousness could be more actively expressed in dreams.

However we approach the subject of consciousness, there

is little hard factual data. Steven Rose, the English neuro-chemist, has proposed a formula which gives a soft subject the patina of hardness:

$$C = f_1(n)f_2(s)$$

where C = consciousness, f = function, n = neuron and s = synapse or connectivity.

In words: Consciousness equals the functions of all otherwise uncommitted neurons multiplied by the number of connections made by these neurons. The word, 'uncommitted' refers to neurons not engaged in seeing or movement, for example, but who is to say that these committed neurons are not also involved in the sensing of self? Thus, it is always 'I' who observe you. According to the formula, however, a very large number comes out to equal consciousness, but it tells us nothing at all about what it is, how it works or what it does.

Writing of self-awareness or self-esteem, the first American psychologist, William James, set down another formula:

$$\text{Self-esteem} = \frac{\text{Success}}{\text{Pretensions}}$$

James's formula surely describes the psychological content of one aspect of consciousness.

In a scientific paper published in 1979, three American neuropsychologists, J. E. LeDoux, D. H. Wilson and M. S. Gazzaniga, equate consciousness with the control and prevention of schizophrenia-like conditions:

Could it be that in the developing organism a constellation of mental systems exists, each with its own values and response probabilities? Then, as maturation continues, the behaviours that these separate systems emit are monitored by the one system we come to use more and more, namely, the verbal, natural language system. Gradually, a concept of self-content develops such that the verbal self comes to know some (though surely not all) of the impulses for action that arise from the other selves, and it tries either to inhibit these impulses or free them, as the case may be. Indeed, it could be argued that the process of psychological maturation in our culture is largely the process through which the verbal system learns to regulate, in accordance with social standards, the behavioural impulses of the many selves that develop inside us.

If consciousness is looked upon in this way, as a symbolic entity whose unique role is unification of separate systems into the self, it may be possible to find an example as an illustration. Here is an old trick which quite plainly demonstrates the recruitment of additional neurons.

Game 3.10: Ask four people to lift you by placing only one index finger each under your armpits and the backs of your knees. At first, they will laugh at you, but try to talk them into it. Tell them to imagine that you are becoming lighter all the time. You may have to fall back on some verbal pyrotechnics in order to sell them the idea, but the better your salesmanship, the more likely they are to succeed. Use whatever magic formulas or mumbo-jumbo you think may hold their attention. If you do the job right, they will be able to lift you using only one index finger each.

This is not a case of mind over matter, but it is evidence that the power of words helps to organize even physical power. Your index finger can be made into a rigid lever, and a little test with a heavy table will show you it can do an amazing amount of work. Your friends will lift you because they themselves believe they can and somehow excite neurons in their spinal cords, called anterior horn cells, in very large numbers. The anterior horn cells recruit many more muscle components in the lifting process.

Whatever consciousness is, it exists in a physical entity which it serves by increasing adaptability and enhancing the chance of survival.

4 Intelligence

There is a charming story about a schools inspector in the old Austro-Hungarian Empire who had called at a one-room village school in the course of his round. He found the teacher helpful and in command, the school room neat and tidy, and the children clean and alert. He was pleased, too, as they answered his test questions correctly, and he ended his examination by asking one more question: 'How many hairs are there on a horse?'

A small, bright-eyed nine-year-old promptly replied, '3,571,962.'

'How do you know?' asked the inspector.

'If you don't believe me,' replied the child, 'count them yourself.'

The inspector was delighted. He assured the teacher that he would tell the story to entertain his colleagues, and he gave the school the highest marks.

A year later, the inspector returned to the village school. After his inspection, which proved quite as satisfactory as it had the year before, the teacher took the liberty of asking if the inspector had told the story of the number of hairs on a horse to his colleagues.

'I did intend to,' the official condescended to reply. 'A very good story it is, indeed. Such a clever child. But, you see, I was not able to tell my colleagues. I simply could not remember the correct number of hairs.'

Whatever you may think of his sense of humour, you will agree that the inspector rather missed the point. Like so many people one knows, he did his job well enough but showed surprising stupidity about all the ordinary things you and I do so well. If he had lost his job or been promoted out of his niche, he might have done rather badly, lacking the ability to adapt to the unusual. His wise superiors had no doubt perceived his limitations and had left him to grow old as a schools inspector.

The bright child, on the other hand, showed no such limitations. Edward de Bono calls the art of stepping outside usual thought patterns 'lateral thinking'. The Gestalt psychologist, Max Wertheimer, who told the story about the schools inspector, called it 'productive thinking'. Wertheimer illustrated productive thinking by means of a game that you can play with your friends.

Game 4.1: Suspend a mirror so that it swings freely. Shine a light so that the mirror reflects the beam on to a scale marked as follows:

$$^+ \quad 5 \quad 4 \quad 3 \quad 2 \quad 1 \quad 0 \quad 1 \quad 2 \quad 3 \quad 4 \quad 5 \quad ^-$$

The actual length of the scale and the size of the numbers will depend on the distance you arrange between it and the mirror. Adjust the scale so that as the mirror swings around, the light moves across the scale evenly, say from -3 to $+3$. Ask your subjects to observe this movement. Now, ask your subjects to turn around or to leave the room. Move the scale so that the light moves from, say -5 to $+1$, that is, through the same degree of arc. Obscure one side of the scale with a card or piece of paper; for example, use the card to cover the half of the scale for $0+$ so that the light falls on the cover rather than on that half of the scale. Your subjects can now look again. Ask each of them where the light now falls on that part of the scale which you have obscured. If you have moved the scale so as to catch the light from the mirror between -5 and $+1$, you will hear various answers. They may range from $+5$, because the observer sees that the light begins at -5 and recalls that it originally moved between -3 and $+3$, to the correct answer, $+1$. The actual correct number is not really important, but ask each subject to explain his answer. To you, the explanation will seem perfectly obvious, of course, but you may be surprised how few of your subjects get it right.

Lateral or productive thinking – or just plain thought – is hard work. As any teacher knows, the results improve with practice though the process of thought seldom gets any easier. Human thought improves with practice in part at least because the person becomes more adept at manipulating symbols. Thus, the arithmetic functions – addition, subtraction, multiplication, division – can all be practised to advantage. What is less clear and therefore more controversial is the degree to which one thinking skill helps another. Do good arithmetic skills help the student to solve problems in the calculus or to reach decisions in parliamentary politics? People seem to accept that a great painter is not likely to be competent in neurobiology although the digital skill of a surgeon may help make him adept at playing a violin. From the standpoint of machinery, digital skills can be tracked down to one part of the brain, the cerebellum. It is possible to believe that fingers trained to move with precision will do well both with a scalpel and with a bow because the cerebellar neurons have learned, but no such centre can be identified for arithmetic skills. There seems to be no physiological reason for assuming that arithmetic skills can be transferred.

Game 4.1 with the mirror and the light involves no specific learning and implies that thought and learning can be distinguished. Perhaps the ability for thought is inherited while skills are learned. The evidence is controversial and incomplete, but you may be able to observe the thought process independent of learning.

Game 4.2: Select two of your friends who are roughly matched in family background and education. Siblings might do, but both would have to be scientists, for example, rather than one a scientist and the other an historian. Explain that you are going to give them a simple problem. Not only do you want a solution, but you want each of them independently to talk to you as he seeks the solution, describing his mental processes. Once they have agreed to the rules of this game, take one friend aside and present the problem. Any problem will do. For example, two rugby teams have played and won the same number of games. 'A' has thirty-two goals and has given away twelve. 'B' has twenty-four goals and has given away ten. Which team leads the other if goal difference is taken into consideration? (The answer, of course, is 'A'.) Take notes on the reply. You are really concerned with the clarity of the explanation, its simplicity and speed. Repeat the process with your second friend. See if you can observe any differences in their explanations. Did you follow essentially the same steps in solving the problem (assuming that you did not use the one suggested)?

There may well be some differences among the verbal skills of your two friends and yourself. Nevertheless, a person who reports his mental steps clearly and succinctly is probably thinking more clearly than one who is less able to explain his thinking.

II

The ability to think and the skills involved in specific kinds of behaviour are components of intelligence. Most modern authorities avoid a definition of the word, though. Too much argument surrounds every attempt to define intelligence. Too little is known about how its attributes come to exist in the machinery of the brain. People who write about intelligence often meet the problem by defining it in terms of the scores on intelligence tests. This is called an operational definition because it derives entirely from the measurement of the trait in operation. It is a kind of definition which is entirely justified within its limits. The same can be said about any definition. I would be right to define sex, for example, as a chromosomal difference leading to the development of physical characteristics which enable male and female to reproduce, but this correct operational description is irrelevant if not useless for understanding the role of sex in society. The socially-dangerous misuse of intelligence test results make it clear that an operational definition may not meet all needs. Before we examine intelligence tests, therefore, I want to consider another attribute which most people would include within the meaning of the word.

Intelligence requires a kind of adaptability. Physical adaptability is exemplified by the changes in blood flow that cause the body to disperse heat when it is hot and to retain heat when it is cold. Intelligence is mental adaptability, that aspect of mind that enables you and me to adapt successfully to new or unusual circumstances. Suppose there is a fire when you are sleeping in a room on the top floor of a hotel. You may be better advised to get out over the roof than to try the more usual means of the staircase if it is crowded or dangerous. Intelligence enables you to make such an important decision correctly in terms of the conditions that you have observed and of what you have learned about fires and crowds.

In the language of Charles Darwin: the more adaptable an organism, the better its chances of selection and the better the survival chance of the individual. Thus, the concept 'intelligence' includes the notion of a goal – the general goal of survival.

Everyday goals, like everyday tests of intelligence, are not usually so grand. Goals direct behaviour at all levels of life. Your goal may be the post office. You want to post a letter because you are hoping it will get you a better job. Psychologists like to talk about drives or motivations, and there is more on this subject in Chapter 9. Suffice it to say, non-goal-directed behaviour lacks coherence and integrity. Intelligence supplies goals.

Game 4.3: For this experiment, you will need a friend's help on two separate occasions. Tell your friend that you are going to time his performance on both occasions. You will need a stopwatch, or a watch with a sweep second hand, but the time of performance is a blind. You will be interested primarily in observing the way your friend works on each occasion.

You will also need two bookshelves, one empty and the other filled with a variety of thirty or forty books. They should be arranged at random. On the first occasion, ask your friend to move the books to the empty shelf and to arrange them by subject and by author within subject as quickly as possible. On the second occasion, perhaps the next day, ask your friend to move the books in any order from one shelf to the empty shelf and back again 10 times. Again, he is to work as quickly as possible.

Your friend has agreed to help you in the interests of science and will no doubt be polite, but it should become obvious soon after he starts the second chore that he finds it far less meaningful than the first. Though the task is patently more simple, your friend may actually take longer to complete it. The goal is irrelevant to the task, whereas on the first occasion the goal requires some use of intelligence even if it is trivial.

You may, however, obtain a curious bonus from the second task. Max Wertheimer, on whose research the game is based, noted that during the second task many subjects developed a rhythm and shifted the books with movements like a dance. Perhaps the brain injects a rhythm in an unconscious attempt to add meaning in the form of pattern to an otherwise meaningless exercise.

Between the grand goal of survival and the day-to-day goals of individual jobs lie a large cluster of goals, drives or motivations which are uniquely culture-oriented. For example, getting from New York to London in three hours instead of seven can only be the goal of behaviour in a culture with adequate technology. Achievement of states of suspended animation can only be used to attain happiness in a culture with the religious and mystical beliefs of the Indian subcontinent. In other words, cultures define intelligence in a multitude of subtle directions.

In his autobiography A. R. Luria tells two stories, both of

which may serve as games to be played with young children. When he was a young man, soon after the Russian revolution, Luria travelled to one of the most backward areas of the Soviet Union, Azerbaijan, to study the perceptual behaviour of illiterate, semi-nomadic tribesmen. They had had no experience of an advanced civilization, either eastern or western. They used stone and iron tools to grow some vegetables in infertile land, shepherded flocks, built temporary shelters, recognized a tight clan organization and exhibited other kinds of intelligent behaviour in an isolated, semi-arid region.

Luria and his associates were familiar with the experiments conducted by Gestalt psychologists using educated Western subjects (see Chapter 10). Their results appear to show that people are born with the ability to recognize circles as a geometrical class. Both ● and ○ were classified as circles by the Gestaltist subjects.

Game 4.4: Show the symbols printed above to pre-school children. Ask each child separately what he sees. You may be surprised and, probably, amused by the answers.

Luria showed the two symbols to the peasants, including peasant women who were separated by Moslem custom from the men. They consistently judged ● to be a coin and ○ to be a moon. They knew nothing about an abstract class of circles, but they knew in what ways the symbol pictures might be useful to them.

Game 4.5: Luria also wanted to know how the Azerbaijanian peasants used words expressing abstractions or generalizations when the words applied to real objects. He wrote:
We presented three subjects (1–3) with drawing of an axe, a saw, and a hammer and asked, 'Would you say these things are tools?'
All three subjects answered yes.
'What about a log?'
1 'It also belongs with these. We make all sorts of

things out of logs – handles, doors, and the handles of tools.'

2   'We say a log is a tool because it works with tools to make things. The pieces of logs go into making tools.'

'But', we remarked, 'one man said a log isn't a tool since it can't saw or chop.'

3   'Some crazy fellow must have told you that! After all, you need a log for tools; together with iron it can cut.'

'But I can't call wood a tool?'

3   'Yes, you can – you can make handles out of it.'

'But can you really say wood is a tool?'

2   'It is! Poles are made out of it, handles. We call all the things we have need of "tools".'

'Name all the tools you can.'

3   'An axe, a mosque [light carriage on springs], and also the tree we tether a horse to if there's no pole around. Look, if we didn't have this board here, we wouldn't be able to keep the water in this irrigation ditch. So that's also a tool, and so is the wood that goes to make a black-board.'

'Name all the tools used to produce things.'

1   'We have a saying: take a look in the fields and you'll see tools.'

3   'Hatchet, axe, saw, yoke, harness, and the thong used in a saddle.'

'Can you really call wood a tool?'

2   'Yes, of course! If we have no wood to use with an axe, we can't plough and we can't build a carriage.'

You may find that you get very much the same kinds of responses from pre-school children when you show them pictures of an axe, a saw and a hammer and ask the same questions. That is not to say that the peasants above were 'childlike', but rather that pre-school children, being relatively unsocialized, see symbols in terms of real things they know rather than as abstract classes of things.

Luria concluded:

Words for these people had an entirely different function from the function they have for educated people. They were used not to codify objects into conceptual schemes but to establish the practical interrelations among things.

When our subjects had acquired some education and had participated in collective discussions of vital social issues, they readily made the transition to abstract thinking. New experiences and new ideas change the way people use language so that words become the principal agent of abstraction and generalization.

From the standpoint of a vague general concept like intelligence, these elegant demonstrations show that the role of culture impinges on every form of voluntary behaviour. How thoughtful, skilful and adaptive Luria's peasant subjects were to the circumstances of their lives. The people who create intelligence tests uphold their universal applicability by pointing to the refinements that have been made over the decades since the tests were first introduced. They point out, for example, that a Chinese subject writes his answers with a brush if he wishes to rather than with the western pen or pencil. The test-makers have indeed overcome such extreme evidence of cultural chauvinism, but it is open to question whether educated, scientifically-oriented research workers are the best judges of their own success in drawing up tests suitable for people who are as different from them as Professor Luria's illiterate peasants.

The importance of any failure by the test-makers is starkly revealed when the people who define intelligence operationally in terms of tests try to extend test results into realms beyond the classroom. They go wrong when they talk about the racial differences in intelligence based on statistics drawn from intelligence tests.

Here are four of the kinds of problems that are put. (For answers see p. 84.)

Game 4.6: Which of these is different?

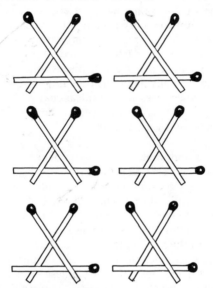

Game 4.7: Arrange these in order of length, starting with the shortest.

$\frac{1}{4}$ inch
1 millimetre
30 centimetres
1 inch
1 kilometre
1 centimetre
1 metre
1 yard
24 millimetres
1 mile
1 foot

Game 4.8: Which of these numbers – 182, 541, 360, 298, 433 – comes next in the sequence?

123   412   323   513   631   ——

Game 4.9: These words all have something in common. What is it?

EFFENDI
ELLEN
ESSAY
EXCEL
SEEDY
CUTIE

These examples were selected because they are reasonably simple, and they are designed to test your ability to solve problems rather than your memory or your skill at a job. They are meant to be solved by people such as you and me who have been educated in technically-advanced western culture. If you accept that someone from an entirely different culture, however, might reply to the question in Game 4.6, 'None of them is wrong', what kind of a problem might you put in place of this one that would be comparable?

Games 4.6 to 4.9 illustrate convergent questions, those which have only one correct answer. Many intelligence tests also contain divergent questions which have more than one answer.

Game 4.10: Think of uses for newspapers and list as many as you can.

According to one textbook, young blacks from American cities did better at this test than any other American social group because for the poor, newspapers substitute as blankets and as paper towels for wiping up spilled heating paraffin.

Answers to Games 4.6 to 4.9

4.6: C. The horizontal match should be placed *over* the first match.

4.7: 1 millimetre, $\frac{1}{4}$ inch, 1 centimetre, 24 millimetres (2.4 centimetres), 1 inch (2.5 centimetres), 30 centimetres, 1 foot (30.4 centimetres), 1 yard, 1 metre (39.4 inches), 1 kilometre, 1 mile (1609 metres).

4.8: 182. The figures in the first number – 123 – add up to 6. The figures in the second number – 412 – add up to 7. The figures in the third number – 323 – add up to 8. The figures in the fourth number – 513 – add up to 9. The figures in the fifth number – 613 – add up to 10. Therefore, the figures in the next number should add up to 11, and 182 is the only number that satisfies this requirement.

4.9: Phonetically, they can all be spelled by letters. Effendi – F N D, Ellen – L N, essay – S A, excel – X L, seedy – C D, cutie – Q T.

Here is another divergent question.

Game 4.11: List all the ways in which you think this product could be improved.

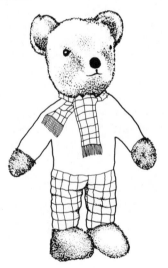

Clearly, Games 4.10 and 4.11 are highly culture-oriented, but they touch on that elusive aspect of intelligence illustrated by the story of the schools inspector. It might also be called creativity.

The term Intelligence Quotient, or IQ, is actually part of the test development process. The first tests were created by two French psychologists, Simon and Binet, who collaborated early in this century. By giving their test to hundreds of school children, they were able to remove questions which seemed to be testing something other than intelligence because the answers revealed greater than average variations. By comparing the range of scores for the same age groups, the test-makers worked out statistical average scores. For each age group the average of all scores on all questions in the test was given the arbitrary value of 100. Averages are, of course, quotients; that is, the answer obtained when one figure is divided by another. The average for a group is an IQ of 100. Those who score above the average have an IQ greater than 100, and those below the average, less than 100. Groups can be defined not only by the ages of the participants, but also by their sex, race, income, religion or any combination of parameters, the general term for identifying qualities that individuals share with one another. As the tests have been given to more and more people over the years, they have been constantly refined. Given a clearly-defined set of parameters, they measure the intelligence of any one individual compared to the average for his group.

Game 4.12: The following IQ test was devised by A. E. Davies for British Mensa, the organization for exceptionally bright people. It is much shorter than the usual IQ test and omits such features as divergent questions. You should allow yourself exactly 40 minutes to answer the 80 questions. Be sure to do the test without interruption at one sitting. Use an alarm clock, or ask a friend to time you. It is legitimate for your friend to warn you at 35 minutes.

Test 1

On each line below, underline the two words which mean most nearly the same. Example: person, man, lad, youth
  1 Absurd, logical, preposterous, popular
  2 Receive, deceive, accept, disown
  3 Negligent, unimportant, careless, cautious
  4 Comparable, intricate, comprehensible, understand-able
  5 Conquer, achieve, find, accomplish
  6 Soft, fragile, severed, brittle
  7 Serene, seething, mobility, tranquil
  8 Subservient, menial, manly, morbid
  9 Stupid, idle, activity, inactive
 10 Transient, immutable, transport, momentary

Test 2

Write, at the end of each line below, the number which continues the series. Example: 2, 4, 6 (8)

11	3, 5, 7	(....)	16	2, 3, 5, 8	(....)
12	28, 21, 14	(....)	17	81, 27, 9, 3	(....)
13	3, 7, 11	(....)	18	1, 4, 9, 16	(....)
14	45, 36, 27	(....)	19	3, 6, 5, 10, 9	(....)
15	2, 4, 8, 16	(....)	20	288, 144, 148, 74, 76	(....)

Test 3

In each sentence below two words have changed places with each other: underline each pair of words.

Example: clothes wear men
 21 A is air gas.
 22 Sugar from not obtained is sea water.
 23 Has triangle every three angles.
 24 Making mistakes of a part is human nature.
 25 Of people are worthy intemperate trust.
 26 Any never employ debaters irony.
 27 Envy traits malice are bad and.
 28 Finds the summer one in sparrows in pairs.
 29 Is comprehend cause to to forgive error.
 30 It is other aimless as any as.

Test 4

In each set of six numbers below, each of the three numbers on the bottom line, including the missing number, is formed by starting with the corresponding number on the top line.

In each set, the same method of arithmetic (e.g., adding two or dividing by three) is used to make the numbers on the bottom line. Find what the different rule is for each different set and write in the missing numbers.

1	3	4
2	4	5

Example

3	5	1
5	7	

4	7	9
11	14	

6	3	2
5	2	

12	3	18
4	1	

3	4	7
6	8	

2	9	3
6	27	

24	100	144
6	25	

27	75	9
18	50	

3	7	4
−2	2	

45	24	12
60	32	

Test 5

On each line below write one letter to continue the series.
Example: AA BB CC D(D)

41	AXY BXY CXY	(....)
42	FEDCB	(....)
43	ECDDCEBF	(....)
44	ABBCBDEFBGHI	(....)
45	DVCWBX	(....)
46	GRCDEGRFGGRH	(....)
47	BHCDGEFGFHIJ	(....)
48	ADGBEHCF	(....)
49	LOMPN	(....)
50	CDECGHIHKLMM	(....)

Test 6

Example: '*Up* is to *down* as *above* is to *below*.' This example is a complete analogy. In each analogy below the third and fourth of the main words are missing and you have to select from the group of words on the right the missing words. In each case underline the two words needed to complete the analogy.

Example: up is to down ... <u>above</u>, beyond, near, <u>below</u>

51   Second is to time ... ounce, return, minute, <u>weight</u>
52   Prediction is to future ... past, absence, memory, present
53   Clumsy is to deft ... ugly, clever, awkward, stupid
54   Hook is to eye ... flange, nut, screw, bolt
55   Dynamic is to static ... politic, active, erg, inert
56   River is to brook ... plateau, mountain, hill, hillock, pile
57   Farmer is to vegetable salesman ... cutter, weaver, cloth, tailor, hatter
58   Where is to room ... which, when, there, now, hour
59   More is to again ... often, repeat, continue, time, still
60   Manner is to matter ... say, frown, custom, word, message

Test 7

On each line below, the words run in pairs. Write the missing word at the end of each line to complete the series.

Example: no, never; perhaps, sometimes; yes (always).

61   Line, two; square, four; pentagon   ....
62   Here, now; nowhere, never; there   ....
63   Canoe, paddle; steamer, screw; yacht   ....
64   Taxicab, taxi; luncheon, lunch; blossom   ....
65   Memory, memorize; courage, encourage; guile ....
66   Analysis, analyse; agreement, agree; danger   ....
67   Legal, illegality; ready, unreadiness; illegible   ....
68   Explanatory, explain; breathy, breathe; facile   ....
69   Division, divide; amendment, amend; peril   ....
70   Angry, anger; abstract, abstraction; irate   ....

Test 8

71 How many miles will a plane fly in 7 hours at an average speed of 500 miles per hour?

72 If there are 5 kinds of chocolates what is the least number a child must buy to be sure of at least three of the same kind?

73 If six machines make 1000 boxes in three days, how many machines could make 1000 boxes in half a day?

74 A bin (with all its corners square) holds 400 cubic feet. If the bin is ten feet long and five feet wide, how deep is it?

75 A man spent one-eighth of his money on rent and four times as much on food and clothes. He then had $9 left. How much did he have at first?

76 A ship has food to last her crew of 250 men for six months. How long would it last 600 men?

77 Mick shared five rolls and Will shared three with Tim, who brought no food but paid fifteen cents. They all ate equal amounts. How much should Will get from the fifteen cents?

78 A snail climbed up a twelve-foot wall at a rate of three feet each day, but slipped down two feet each night. How many days did it take him to reach the top?

79 How many miles does a fly travel flying non-stop from end to end of a sixty-foot carriage at sixty miles an hour in a train leaving station A at 6 p.m. and reaching B, 90 miles away, at 9 p.m.?

80 Write the way in which you could arrange three nines to equal eleven.

The correct answers are on pages 90–1. An average adult scores about 20 correct answers! To be eligible for Mensa, you would have to score about 70.

IQ tests do not define what they measure. Nor do they define the groups to which they are administered; that is, it is not possible to work backwards from the test and say, for example, that this particular test result assigns an individual to such-and-such a group (unless the group is identified by test scores, as when all subjects with test scores under 50 regardless of age, sex or any other parameter are classified as Imbeciles).

Within socially-defined groups, racially or otherwise differentiated, the range of intellectual potential is probably about the same. Evidence from comparative studies using intelligence tests suggests that test scores decline as people grow older, but even this decline may be conditioned by social factors; for example, as your school years fade into the past, you may also forget the skill of taking tests – if there is such a skill!

Intelligence tests are useful because they prove that this trait is a continuum like any other, and they compare the abilities of individuals to do certain jobs. For these reasons, literally hundreds of such tests have been developed. Because of educational differences even within the English-speaking world, tests used in the United States are not suitable for Britain, and so on for other parameters. Through such refinement, intelligence tests have become subtle and relevant tools for the operational definition of this trait. They have come no closer to identifying the physiological machinery of intelligence, however. For this, we must first find out what memory is, and how we learn.

Answers to IQ Test

1	absurd preposterous	14	18
2	receive accept	15	32
3	negligent careless	16	12
4	comprehensible understandable	17	1
5	achieve accomplish	18	25
6	fragile brittle	19	18
7	serene tranquil	20	38
8	subservient menial	21	a air
9	idle inactive	22	from is
10	transient momentary	23	has every
11	9	24	of is
12	7	25	of intemperate
13	15	26	any debaters

27	traits and	54	nut bolt
28	finds in	55	active inert
29	is to	56	mountain hillock
30	other [the 2nd] as	57	weaver tailor
31	3	58	when hour
32	1	59	repeat continue
33	14	60	word message
34	16	61	five
35	6	62	then
36	9	63	sail
37	36	64	bloom
38	− 1	65	beguile
39	6	66	endanger
40	16	67	legibility
41	D	68	facilitate
42	A	69	imperil
43	A	70	ire
44	J	71	3500
45	A	72	11
46	G	73	36
47	K	74	8
48	I	75	24
49	Q	76	$2\frac{1}{2}$
50	O	77	1
51	ounce weight	78	10
52	past memory	79	180
53	clever stupid	80	$\frac{99}{9}$

5 Memory

I

Push aside the everyday word 'memory', and think for a moment about what it is. Not just that you can remember your name and a lot more besides, or that someone may dramatically 'lose' his memory, but what must happen to allow you to remember and to call up from memory. Almost certainly, some fairly permanent physical change must occur, presumably in nerve cells, when new data is learned.

No one yet knows what those changes are. We do know 'that together with scar tissue,' as the British neurochemist, Steven Rose, has written, 'memories are the most durable environmentally important individual characteristic.'

There are two kinds of memory: short- and long-term. They are sequential. Short-term memory apparently must precede long-term, but long-term memory does not necessarily succeed short-term.

Game 5.1: To play this game, you need a pencil. Read through the list of words just once at normal speed. Do not study it or attempt to memorize the words. As soon as you have read it through, turn the page and write down as many words as you can remember in any order that you recall them:

earth	life	lock	apple
dog	shape	pill	wall
peach	spine	tank	saw
ball	brick	thing	field
flower	cat	door	potato
follow	cow	Maharishi	lamp

When you have written all the words you can remember, compare your list with the one above. You should find two words or groups of words near the top of your list. The last word, lamp, and possibly the word or two before it should be followed by the word, Maharishi, and possibly the words on either side of it. The order may be different, but the reasons why these words appear near the top of your list illustrates the nature of short-term memory. It contains data specified by two criteria, recency and importance. Importance is represented by Maharishi, the only proper noun and the only noticeably foreign word. The last words in the list are of course the most recent. If you have recalled the words on either side of Maharishi, it is probably because you paid extra attention to them in light of the importance you assigned to the unusual word.

The so-called primacy-recency effect illustrated by Game 5.1 is also called the von Restorff effect after the German psychologist who described it. The von Restorff effect can draw in words on either side of the important word, as we have seen, but much of what happens around us never gets as far as short-term memory because we do not notice it.

Game 5.2: Tap your fingers gently against your arm. The feel of it remains for a moment, but then there is only a recollection which fades rapidly.

Game 5.3: Ask someone to tap a knife or a nail on a hard surface or to whistle briefly. Close your eyes to listen. Again, note how the distinctness of the tone fades.

Game 5.4: Close your eyes. Open them very briefly and close them again. Notice how quickly the sharp image fades.

Game 5.5: Stare straight ahead. Wave a pencil or your finger back and forth in front of your eyes. You should see a shadowy image on your left when the pencil moves to the right and vice versa. To maintain a continuous image without a shadow, you have to move the pencil through 10 cycles, or 20 times in 5 seconds.

All of these sensory experiences illustrate how sensation provides a sort of anteroom out of which short-term memory may open, but the fading recollections of the last four games are not retained. If you doubt this, read on for a page or two and then try to remember the games. You paid attention to the images but probably not to remembering them.

The attention factor has obvious survival value. Either we know what is important to us or we learn about it. We remember that and forget the rest.

Game 5.6: Ask a friend to be the subject for this demonstration. Select any three letters and say them aloud slowly, then straight away ask your friend to count backward by threes from 100. After 20 seconds, ask him to repeat the letters. There is a good chance he will have forgotten them.

Your friend has heard the three letters, but you have redirected his attention, destroying any short-term memory that may have begun to form.

Try Game 5.6 with any three short words. Your friend may find recall much easier. Each of the words represents an important kind of chunking, the grouping together of sensations into a pattern. Short-term memory seems to work better, or to encompass more material, when it is chunked. Words withstand the deflection of attention perhaps because of their associations or meanings.

Chunking was illustrated in 1887 by an English psychologist, Joseph Jacobs, who used this test:

Game 5.7: Again you will need a friend to act as your subject. Prepare a list of two-digit numbers. Read aloud any four of the numbers, about one a second, and ask the subject to repeat them. Now read five different numbers and ask the subject to repeat them. Now read six numbers, have them repeated, and so on up to ten numbers.

You should find that your friend will be able to repeat each group of numbers correctly until you read him eight or more. Then he will make mistakes. If you use letters instead of numbers, your subject may be able to repeat up to seven correctly, but if you replace the letters with three-letter words, he may be able to repeat only six correctly. Note, however, that six three-letter words include eighteen letters!

When he tried his test on children, Joseph Jacobs found that short-term memory span increased to six, seven or eight as the children grew older. Indeed, this improvement with age is so regular that the test still forms a part of the Binet intelligence tests. Inability to recall the chunk of six, seven or eight items is often an indication of mental deficiency, but a greater recall span does not reflect higher intelligence. George A. Miller, an American psychologist, refers to this phenomenon as 'the magic number seven, plus or minus two', so regular is it.

There appears to be one form of short-term memory which escapes the rule of seven plus or minus two.

Game 5.8: You will need either several hundred pictures cut from magazines or catalogues, or two fat magazines of similar date and content. You will also need a subject. If you are using pictures, hand your friend about 100. He is to look at each one and give it a name related to its content. It is best if he says the name aloud, but do not comment or stop for discussion. He can take his time as long as he moves right along without going back to any picture. When the subject has finished, take twenty of the pictures he has seen and mix them with twenty new ones. Ask the subject to sort them into pictures he has seen before and new ones. He will make very few mistakes. If you are using two magazines, ask the subject to thumb through one and then through the second. When he starts on the *second*, ask him to tell you after he has finished how many of the ads in the second magazine also appeared in the first. He is not to count aloud or on his fingers. Again, he should make few mistakes.

The conclusion must be that visual memory is stronger than memory based on other sensations. Whether this is because of something inherent in vision – for example, its importance to humans – or because the pictures all have important associations, it is not possible to say.

II

There is a simple game that reveals clearly the distinction between short- and long-term memory. It was published in 1962 by an American psychologist, B. B. Murdock, Jr.

Game 5.9: Make up a list of twenty common words. Read them to a friend at about one word per second. As soon as you have finished, ask your friend to write down all the words he can remember in any order.

Like your own response to Game 5.1, your subject will probably begin with the last three or four words in your list. Now, if there was a straightforward positional memory decline – that is, if the further back in the list the word fell, the less likely you would be to remember it – you might be dealing with a single form of memory. That this is not the case is revealed by the fact that most people also recall the first two or three words in the list. If their recall is charted, it looks like Figure 5.1.

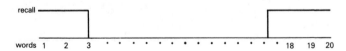

Fig. 5.1: Linear representation of recall in Game 5.9

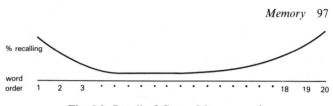

% recalling

word
order   1   2   3   · · · · · · · · · · · · · ·   18   19   20

Fig. 5.2: Recall of Game 5.9 as a graph

Most authorities agree that the ability to recall the first words in the list is evidence of a second kind of memory.

Based in part on Murdock's experiment, it is possible to begin to assign some time periods to the different kinds of memory. Sensory awareness, the anteroom to memory, may last about fifteen seconds. Short-term memory may exist from about fifteen seconds up to five or ten minutes, depending on the kind of experience. Anything longer than about ten minutes is long-term memory. Using your twenty-word list and a stopwatch, however, you can time Game 5.9 from the moment you begin to read the list to the time when your friend finishes writing the words he can recall. It will come to about a minute. If the phenomenon represented by the recall of the first two or three words is long-term memory, then according to this test it comes into existence more rather than less rapidly. The timing is of particular interest when we examine the physical bases of memory.

As with short-term memory, relevance determines the selection of what goes into long-term memory. Relevance is an individual matter, depending on the personality and situation of the subject, but you can suggest to yourself how it works by experimenting with a technique called shadowing. In shadowing, one listens to and repeats one message while also listening to a second message.

Game 5.10: You will need three friends to help you with this experiment, two men and one woman or two women and one man. Assign yourself the role of subject. One friend should sit directly to your right and another to your left at the same distance. Let us call you, the subject, A, the two people of the same sex, B and C, and the person of the opposite sex, D. D will be in a position to change places easily with either B or C, thus:

B ◄———— 3ft ————► A ◄———— 3ft ————► C (D)

B reads aloud flatly and evenly from a text. A repeats each word or brief phrase as B reads. Practise this for a while. Then, C begins to read a list of random words. C should also read flatly and evenly. A must try to attend to C while shadowing B; that is, while repeating what B reads. During the experiment, with as little warning or movement as possible, D's voice should replace C's and continue to read the list of random words. It will also be interesting if C or D can change languages once during the experiment, continuing to read random words flatly and evenly. This shift too should be accomplished without warning. All of you should agree in advance to a time limit for the experiment, for example, five minutes.

The results are usually as follows: A remembers whether C (D) is present or not, can tell if C changes from a man's to a woman's voice or vice versa, and notices special signals from C (D) such as a whistle. A does not remember the content of C's (D's) message, recognize the language of the message, note whether the language changes during the experiment, or distinguish words from nonsense syllables. In other words, without attention, or relevance as defined in this game, long-term memory for spoken language is not formed.

Like short-term memory, moreover, long-term memory improves if data is presented in chunks. This is true of events composed of many sensations just as it applies to learning abstract data such as language. Everyone has experienced recall triggered by a song or a smell. A scene, even an entire period in one's life, springs to mind when the appropriate trigger is pressed. Presumably, the memory consists of the trigger sensation plus all of its other parts. In theory, any other segment of the memory could act as trigger with the same efficacy. Perhaps you will have experienced the recall of a single memory on two different occasions by two different sensory elements, for example, a colour and a touch sensation.

Game 5.11: It is hard to experiment with the chunking represented by natural events, but the abstract kind can be illustrated. Again, you will want the help of a friend. Write down the following list of words on a piece of paper.

no	no	yes
no	yes	no
no	no	yes
yes	no	no
no	yes	yes
no	yes	yes
yes	yes	no

Ask your friend to study the list for five minutes. Time him, and then take the list away. Ask him to repeat it exactly. The probability is that after eight or nine items, he will make mistakes. The length of the study period should make little difference.

Now, give your friend the following list, written on a second sheet of paper.

$$no - no - no = 0$$
$$no - no - yes = 1$$
$$no - yes - no = 2$$
$$no - yes- yes = 3$$
$$yes - no - no = 4$$
$$yes - no - yes = 5$$
$$yes - yes - no = 6$$
$$yes - yes - yes = 7$$

Ask him to study the list. Fix the period of study anywhere between five and thirty minutes. Tell the subject that you are going to read this list of words. He is to group them into threes, recode each group of three as a number and write down the number. Read the words slowly and evenly. Do not read them in groups of three.

The chances are that the subject will remember all eight numbers. In other words, he will have remembered twenty-one different words in sequence – though not quite the same sequence, as you can see by checking the two lists – as against eight or nine.

It is this same kind of chunking which forms the foundation of all digital computer programs, although only two states may be used instead of three. Each on-off unit is called a 'bit' in information theory. The size of a computer memory is measured by the number of bits it can contain. Thus, in an 'old-fashioned' computer, in which the memory consists of transistors instead of microchip circuits, each transistor may be on or off.

The neuron may also be on or off, and by analogy the memory capacity of your brain can be estimated in bits. The problem here is that there are numerous possibilities for the linking together of neurons which could increase the actual number of bits. Nevertheless, human memory capacity has been estimated at between 10^{11} and 10^{14} bits of information. By comparison, the entire *Encyclopedia Britannica* contains 2×10^8 bits, a far smaller number. Apart from the question of how neurons link together in memory, however, we have not yet dealt with the nature of a memory bit. How much or what kind of an experience causes the neuron to become the reservoir of a bit? What causes the memory switch to turn on, or in other words, what is recall?

Once again, we are interested in physiological machinery. The psychological qualities of long-term memory appear to be remarkably like those of short-term memory. The difference between them appears to be entirely a matter of duration, though short-term memory must also precede long-term. But it is these two distinctions which indicate that separate mechanisms underlie the two psychological aspects of memory.

There is one psychological distinction between them, however, which is worth noting here although it will be described in greater detail in Chapters 6 and 10. The chunking which facilitates long-term memory is also associated with patterns or models of the external world, some of them possibly inborn. These models form the basis of Gestalt psychology and modern Chomskian linguistics. They are interesting now because the models affect long-term memory but apparently have no significance in short-term memory.

III

Amnesia means loss of memory. It may be caused by a blow to the head, by a general shock to the body such as can occur in an automobile accident, or by disease. There are two kinds of amnesia, retrograde and post-traumatic. Retrograde amnesia is the loss of memory before the causative event, the phenomenon much beloved by writers of fiction. Post-traumatic amnesia is memory loss after the causative event. Most amnesia of both kinds is temporary. Rarely does the victim wander the streets of life unable to recall even his own name. In the very few cases of total amnesia, there has usually also been severe permanent brain damage.

Retrograde amnesia slowly disappears with the earliest events returning first, except that the last brief period before the trauma – usually no more than a few seconds – has disappeared forever. People may never remember what they were doing just before a car accident, but they will probably recover the memory, for example, of who was driving.

Post-traumatic amnesia never occurs without retrograde amnesia, but the reverse is not true. If there has been post-traumatic amnesia, memory is spotty rather than consistently lost. Chunks of lost memory return in a jig-saw puzzle fashion, gradually filling in the picture though seldom completing it. Some small segments of the post-injury period may be permanently lost, but they are not consistently those which follow immediately after the trauma. One of the most common kinds of post-traumatic amnesia is seen after sports accidents. For example, a football player suffers a blow causing him to forget both the events leading up to the knock and the goal he kicked immediately afterwards. His amnesia may not even be noticed by his team until minutes later when he runs the wrong way.

Permanent memory loss in amnesia affects short-term memory. This is most obvious in retrograde amnesia because the permanent loss covers only a brief period immediately preceding the trauma. There has not been time for the lost memory to enter a permanent store. The earlier memories return, beginning with the earliest. The trauma can also impair more or less briefly the ability to form new memories, however, and this is post-traumatic amnesia. Probably post-traumatic memory loss is erratic because it depends on the importance of the events to the individual. Thus, the injured football player runs the wrong way but remembers that it is the second half.

An even more blatant form of short-term memory impairment is a sign of the condition called Korsakov's syndrome. The patient suffers no loss of long-term memory. He knows who he is, the members of his family and why he is ill, but if a visitor leaves the room, the patient instantly forgets the visit. The doctor can enter the room three times during a morning and be greeted each time as though it was his first visit. The patient ceases to learn. Korsakov's syndrome is frequently a sign of alcohol poisoning, but it may also signify any damage or disease that produces speech aphasia; that is, the incapacity to speak correctly. In this case the aphasia is caused by damage to the left temporal cortex, one part of the language regulating zone. Indeed, there may be a connection between short-term memory and this brain region. At least, memory formation may require the active participation of this symbolizing zone.

In addition to amnesia and damage in the left temporal region, there are other possible causes of short-term memory impairment. Cannabis users may experience short-term memory loss which disappears when the effect of the drug wears off. Patients given electroconvulsive shock therapy (ECT) often experience a brief amnesic period. Experimental anoxia (oxygen deprivation), chemical convulsants, anesthesia and sudden cooling as well as ECT have been used to shock an animal soon after it has learned a task. If the shock is applied close enough to the training period, the learning disappears. The time interval cannot be fixed accurately, but the shock must occur within minutes. If the interval between training and shock is too long, no memory impairment will be noticed.

It appears that the mechanism of short-term memory is relatively easy to disrupt. The machinery underlying long-term memory is not only less subject to destruction but physically different. The relative speed with which short-term memory comes and goes requires a fast change in neuronal behaviour which is relatively easily reversed. Such a change probably takes place at the synapse. Short-term memory has been attributed to synaptic facilitation, a change in the electrical properties of neurons at the synapse between them which eases the signalling at least temporarily. Thus, attention to a visual signal could engage the necessary visual pathway causing the synaptic changes which embody short-term memory. Conversely, a shock could stop transmission allowing the synapse to return to its pre-excited state. These examples are speculative, of course, but they point to the one mechanism that seems to fit all the facts.

The problem of long-term memory is obviously altogether different. Soon after World War II, the English neuropsychologist, W. Grey Walter, discovered that there was a change in the brain waves near the frontal lobes associated with learning a task. This EEG phenomenon has been tracked down to the hippocampus. Hippocampal neurons may also synthesize a new chemical when long-term memory is in the process of formation; that is, when the experimental animal learns something.

I pointed out in Chapter 2 that it has not been possible

to locate a memory. The Canadian surgeon, Wilder Penfield, succeeded in artificially stimulating recall, but destruction of the brain tissue beneath the microelectrode does not destroy the memory. Long-term memory presents a double problem: what is it and where?

The most likely answer to the what question has seemed to be, a chemical change. Cells are microscopic chemical factories. Cells in the pancreas and the adrenal glands, for example, synthesize hormones. Cells in the lymphatic system manufacture antibodies. Muscle cells lengthen and shorten by alternately breaking and forming chemical bonds between two large protein molecules. All cells synthesize enzymes, the proteins that speed chemical reactions under body conditions. Neurons conduct signals by means of a flow of ions, and transmit signals by means of a chemical which they synthesize and store. Any lasting change in a cell must be embodied in a chemical. A new molecule is formed or an old one destroyed, but whatever the nature of the chemical change, it must last if the behaviour of the cell is to be altered permanently. Thus, long-term memory must be associated with either formation of new molecules or destruction of old ones.

Both the structure and function of a cell are controlled by its genes. Since J. W. Watson and F. H. C. Crick described the probable structure of the DNA molecule in 1953, evidence has accumulated to show that internal control follows a straightforward course dictated by the synthesis of successive molecules. The DNA of the gene directs formation of RNA. RNA in turn directs synthesis of protein. Each gene forms a template for an RNA molecule, and each RNA molecule either acts as a template for one protein or becomes involved in the machinery of protein synthesis. The fundamental sequence is DNA → RNA → protein. Protein molecules express every permanent feature of a cell, both functional, such as the cell's enzymes, and structural. It is reasonable to assume that if long-term memory depends on a permanent chemical change, evidence of it would appear somewhere along this sequence.

The search for a memory molecule began during the late 1950s with a most unlikely experimental animal, the flatworm, planarian. Less than an inch long, these creatures possess an elementary nervous system with a ganglion at the front end that performs primitive co-ordinating functions like a brain. Cut a flatworm in half, moreover, and you get two new individuals. The front half regenerates a tail section and the back half a head. Planaria were taught to avoid light, which usually attracts them, by sending a mild electric current through their bath whenever they approached a light. The trained creatures were cut in half. It was then found that the newly-developed animals from both halves retained the light-avoidance learning. The researchers reasoned that because neurons throughout the body had been altered by the learning process, the chemical change affected all of them. After suitable chemical analysis, they reported that a new kind of RNA had been found in the trained animals.

The results of research into memory molecules have consistently proved extremely hard to reproduce. The first burst of enthusiasm for flatworm RNA fell on ground made stony by questions such as: If there is a new RNA in the trained animals, is it restricted to the nervous system? Might it not also turn up in muscle, for example? And might it not have arisen because of the trauma of being cut in half rather than from the training? Indeed, it was pointed out that the quantity of new RNA is extremely small, and critics wondered whether if it was really present, it might not have been there undetected even before the training. The enthusiastic planaria researchers even published a charming magazine to broadcast their results, but *The Worm Runners' Digest* did not survive the fifties.

Scientists in the United States, the United Kingdom and Sweden moved on from RNA to proteins, using learning in small mammals, chickens and goldfish. Perhaps the most spectacular discovery was reported in 1968 by a group at Houston, Texas, led by Georges Ungar. The group trained rats to fear the dark, a milieu which they normally prefer.

From the brains of the trained animals, they were able to isolate a small protein-like molecule which was not present in untrained rat brains. The scientists injected the chemical into the brains of untrained *mice* and found that these animals too avoided the dark. Having analysed the chemical, the investigators synthesized it in their laboratory. They named it scotophobin (fear of the dark). This artificial molecule was injected into naive rats and mice, and these animals also feared the dark. Although Ungar's findings have never been completely contradicted, similar transfer experiments have failed to sustain the momentum he established. For example, it was found that if material from a trained animal was injected into an untrained animal, the result was usually positive (that is, the injected animal also feared the dark), but if the injected material came from the brains of *two* trained animals, the untrained recipient actually did less well (in learning to fear the dark) than untreated animals.

If the search for a memory molecule has not been abandoned, the early excitement has waned. Not only are there serious procedural and technical problems, but the logic of a scotophobin molecule is tricky to say the least. Is it specifically fear of a certain quality or condition of darkness that is being transferred, or is it a general fear? Is there a molecule for Shakespeare's *Hamlet*, or for the 'To be or not to be' soliloquy? You can appreciate the difficulty.

The notion of a memory molecule may just be naive. Networks of neurons with their thousands of interconnections, some excitatory and some inhibitory, must also play some role in long-term memory.

IV

In order to remember, your brain must first locate the memory. This act of location – remembering – may be accidental, as when a sensation triggers your memory, or it may follow a deliberate search.

Game 5.12: Here are five questions:

1   What was Mozart's telephone number?
2   What was D. H. Lawrence's telephone number?
3   What is the Buckingham Palace telephone number?
4   What is the phone number of your best friend?
5   What is your telephone number?

You will not bother to search for an answer to question 1. Unless you are writing a thesis about Lawrence, you are also unlikely to take question 2 very seriously although it is at least plausible that Lawrence had a phone. You probably do not try to remember the answer to number 3 because you have not learned the number, but a little research in the directory can put that right. Questions 4 and 5 probably draw forth unhesitating responses from your memory.

Game 5.13: Now, call to mind the house in which you grew up. How many windows did it have? Are you sure? If possible, check your memory by going to look at the house or by asking a relative.

Image retrieval can be quite independent of language itself. But where is the picture of your childhood home? It could be filed under 'house, early life in', but it could equally well be distributed so that your own room lives in a slot with a feeling of anger associated with the parental command: 'Go to your room.' Your parents' bedroom, a psychoanalyst might argue, would be recalled if you could resurrect your infantile desire for your opposite-sex parent. The English psychiatrist, Anthony Storr, holds that 'the "tip of the tongue" phenomenon occurs because the brain does not necessarily store the complete letter sequence of every word which the subject can recognize. The words which we know we know but cannot recall are words which have been incompletely stored and which are therefore incompletely known.' But then how do you explain forgetting something you have known well for years? Most of us have experiences like this. We call the wrong child, often all of them, naming last the one we want. We introduce an old friend and forget her name. Is it just because of passing distraction, or was Freud right: slips of the tongue always have an explanation in the unconscious. Possibly, each brain's filing system is unique, an arrangement which could explain the characteristic chaos of one's dreams.

A. R. Luria is the Russian neuropsychologist whose name turns up more than any other in this book because it is primarily his approach to understanding the brain that I am using. Professor Luria wrote a fascinating account, *The Mind of a Mnemonist*, about one of his patients who had a prodigious memory. 'S' made his living as a vaudeville act. He could remember long lists of words or numbers read to him just once. His was a peculiarly barren skill though, because his memory was inefficient with ordinary textual material like this paragraph. The content would get in the way of his peculiar memory system. 'S' had wanted to be a musician, but music caused him to see swirls of colour so bright and continuous that it got in the way of the notation itself. His memory was embodied in imagery.

Though he did not know it, 'S' used an ancient memory system called mnemotechnics. The mnemonist takes the image of a scene containing a logical sequence of places, for example, the houses on a street, real or imaginary, or the furniture and ornaments in a room, and he places the words he wants to recall in association with the objects. Thus, 'S' would hear a list of words beginning: horse, train, sick, throng, divide, roseate, and so on. He would visualize a street of houses, each with its peculiar shape, colour and size. 'Horse' would be assigned to the big blue house, first on the left; 'train' to the large modern house opposite; 'sick' to the small white cottage next door to that. ... When 'S' wanted to recall the list of words, he walked down the street in his imagination and picked the words off the houses. You can understand how hard it was for 'S' to remember a textual passage containing a logic of its own, but the Greek and medieval mnemonists who lived before the invention of printing taught themselves whole speeches in this manner.

Game 5.14: You can learn to use mnemotechnics. You can use a street or a room, but you may find the image of the clothes rack easier to begin with. Imagine a pole consisting of numbers on which are hangers consisting of rhyming words. Over the word-hangers are hung items of clothing; that is, the words you want to remember.

Pole:	1	2	3	4	5	6
Hanger:	bun	shoe	tree	door	hive	sticks
Item:	horse	train	sick	throng	divide	roseate

Now, how is one to associate the item with the rhyming hanger? Well, the horse is a sausage inside a bun. 'Shoe train' becomes its own image. Similarly, a sick tree and a throng in front of a door are clear images. Divide and hive share an internal rhyme, or you can picture a bee keeper dividing a hive. When they are burning, sticks cast a roseate light.

Perhaps the pole with its rhyming hangers is enough help, but rhyming also plays a role in saws such as: '"i" before "e" except after "c" or when sounding like "a" as in neighbour or weight.' And, 'Thirty days hath September, April, June and November/All the rest have thirty-one/ Excepting February alone/Which hath but twenty-eight days clear/And twenty-nine in each leap year.' In saws such as these, rhyming is a form of chunking which makes the material easier to get at.

Another useful saw – for speliologists and others interested in stalactites and stalagmites: 'When tites come down, mites go up.'

Mnemonics can be used for much more *recherché* subjects. Physiologists who must know the names of the nerves that pass through the superior orbital foramen (one of the natural openings) of the skull try to remember: 'Lazy French tarts lie naked in anticipation.' From this elegant expression, they hope to recall: lacrimal, frontal, trochlear, lateral, nasociliary, internal, abducens.

Game 5.15: Here is another mnemonic system you might like to try. It involves the use of numbers to recall letters and form words or parts of a word – enough to stand for the whole word. First, you have to memorize the number alphabet. It is built up on the principal of sound similarities.

1	has one downstroke	t	d	th
2	has two downstrokes	n		
3	has three downstrokes	m		
4	last letter of four	r		
5	Roman for 50	l		
6	j is the mirror image of 6	j	sh	ch
7	two sevens back to back: ⅄	k	g(hard)	
8	f in script resembles 8	f	v	
9	reversal, rotated: ℗	p	b	
10	zero	z	s	

Note that rather like Arabic script, this alphabet contains no vowels.

Thus, from our previous list:

horse	40
train	142
sick	07
throng	147
divide	181
roseate	401

Or, 695 = ch (a) p (e) l

Games 5.14 and 15 demonstrate one obvious fact about retrieval: the more associations with which you can surround a memory, the better your chances of recalling it. These useful associations are probably emotional as well as perceptual and intellectual. That is no doubt why one never forgets one's own name while in normal health.

Perhaps for most of us, the role of associations becomes more clear as we grow older. Common observation suggests that old people remember past events more efficiently than recent ones. In part, this weakness may be a failure of the transfer machinery that carries a memory from short- to long-term store. Except in cases of degenerative brain diseases, old people display no significant impairment of short-term memory. Possibly, the decline in their ability to recall new events is due to weakening of the recall mechanism itself. On the other hand, memory for new data in the aged, as in the rest of us, improves if the data fit into a context supplied by existing memory. A mathematician finds his memory for new mathematical techniques much more efficient than his memory for current political affairs, let us say. Women who have raised children, superintended weddings and helped with the grandchildren may well remember the details of recent family happenings more clearly than their husbands. Indeed, older people who give up on their memories do so at their own peril. They are themselves often largely to blame if they feel that their memory is declining. If you say, for example, that you cannot remember such terms as neuron, action potential or transmitter, of course you will not. Just like ordinary schooling, always a difficult chore for most of us, memory requires effort. The older you are, the more effort perhaps, but because one is older, one ought to know some memory tricks the young have still to learn. For example, it is always a good crutch to memory if you write something down.

Experiments using small doses of drugs thought to assist memory have been tried with groups of old people. In almost every trial, the results have been positive, but similar trials with younger people fail to show the same results. Probably because the old people being tested are institutional patients in most cases, the extra attention given them by the research workers explains the improvement in their ability to learn. If this is true, it is a good example of scientific neglect of the obvious. Everyone has noticed that, old or young, we learn more quickly from attentive teachers.

Yet when all is said and done, old people do gradually lose the ability to remember new things. Until we know more about the machinery of memory, the causes of its decline will remain obscure.

Perhaps one of the most useful models of memory incorporating the available data has been proposed by the British neuroanatomist, J. Z. Young. According to Young, memory is not just a matter of learning by opening up pathways; it is equally the evidence of shutting them down. Memory requires inhibition as well as facilitation. Based on his research with the octopus, Young has suggested that there is a basic memory unit. In Figure 5.3, the memory unit contains instructions either to retreat from or to attack an object which may be either painful or edible (though it could contain two sets of instructions of a quite different kind).

The classifying neuron responds to a sensation, say a taste. It has two outputs: one produces an attack and the other, retreat. Suppose the animal tries to eat the object but receives a painful stimulus. The retreat output cell then inhibits the attack output cell. Inhibition could be produced by the synthesis in the cell of a new chemical because Young's model proposes that memory reflects permanent inhibition. It also suggests that once the inhibition is established, forgetting becomes impossible. Young has said: 'I don't believe in forgetting.' This being true, failure to recall would

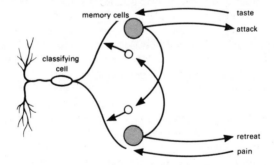

Fig. 5.3: A model of a memory system in the octopus

occur only when the inhibited circuit could not be located by the recall mechanism. It could be argued that conditioning experiments show that a conditioned response can be erased (see Chapter 6), but this is not what is usually meant by forgetting.

Where are these memory units, and how could you lose one? As one is yet to be found, even in the octopus brain, there is no answer. A physical discovery, holography, has been enlisted to suggest what could happen in recall. A hologram is a photograph taken with laser light in such a way that the illumination of any part of the plate causes the whole picture to reappear. You can understand how recall triggered by a smell or a sound seems to be an analogy. Thus, if a memory is a widely-distributed sequence of memory units consisting of sensed items – light level, colour, smell, and so on – recall would require a sort of laser beam flashing through the brain to reassemble the bits. Unfortunately, there is no obvious analogy for the laser beam in the brain.

Analogies like holography and the popular computer image of brain function can suggest avenues for research, but they must not be taken too literally. Machine memory, for example, is phenomenal especially since the invention of the microchip, but there is no reason to assume that machine and human memory operate in the same way. A rigid adherence to analogy could actually slow the search for the machinery of living memory as well as our understanding of the nature of learning.

6 Learning

I

Jean Piaget, the Swiss developmental psychologist, based much of his original theory on observations of his own son, Laurent. This is how he described Laurent's acquisition of one skill:

> At 16 months, 5 days, Laurent is seated before a table and I place a bread crust in front of him, out of reach. Also to the right of the child I place a stick about 25 cm long. At first Laurent tries to grasp the bread without paying any attention to the instrument, and then he gives up....
>
> I then put the stick between him and the bread; it does not touch the objective but nevertheless carries with it an undeniable visual suggestion. Laurent again looks at the bread, without moving, looks very briefly at the stick, then suddenly grasps it and directs it towards the bread. But he grasped it toward the middle and not at one of the ends so that it is too short to obtain the objective. Laurent then puts it down and resumes stretching out his hand towards the bread. Then, without spending much time on this movement, he takes up the stick again, this time at one of its ends (chance or intention?), and draws the bread to him.... Two successive attempts yield the same result.
>
> An hour later I place a toy in front of Laurent (out of his reach) and a new stick next to him. He does not even try to catch the object with his hand; he immediately grasps the stick and draws the toy to him.

Thanks in large part to Piaget, the study of learning today devotes much time to the development of the infant. The human infant grows into the human adult for better or for worse, whereas the rat – for decades the favourite experimental animal of the behaviourists – remains a rat.

Developmental psychologists have been able to show that before it is a month old an infant distinguishes its mother's face from other faces. In less than half that time the infant can distinguish its mother's voice. Infant learning is a two-way street, moreover. The parents learn to understand signs and cries, thus enabling the infant to sharpen and discriminate its own responses. The popular assumption that language evolves out of cries and gurgles is not true because the ability to understand and use language capacity itself appears to mature before the child actually begins to speak. More will be said about language later in this chapter, but these are the kinds of questions that developmental psychology can elucidate.

Piaget showed that the child's comprehension of space and volume are learned. If you have a three-year-old available, try this Piagetian test.

Game 6.1: You will need two glasses or glass vases, one notably short and fat and the other much taller and thinner. Fill the short glass about half full of water while the child is watching you. Now, while he is still watching, pour the water from the first glass into the second. Ask the child which glass contains more water. The chances are he will say 'the second'. Try the same test with a child of five, and he will probably answer that you have just poured the water from one glass to the other so they must have held the same amount.

It is less easy to experiment with your own learning, but the American psychologist, Edward Thorndike, tried this simple test himself.

Game 6.2: Thorndike drew a line exactly four inches long. On a different piece of paper, he drew several lines successively free hand, trying to make each of them four inches long. He measured these lines, noting the results, and then on another piece of paper, drew several more lines. He repeated these steps until his results began to approximate four-inch lines with some regularity.

At first, Thorndike took this result to be a sign of motor learning, and he noted the time needed to acquire the skill. Later, he began to doubt the validity of the experiment. From time to time he repeated the experiment. When no improvement in accuracy took place, as sometimes happened, he reasoned that he had actually been learning to repeat his erroneous lines. Then, he also began to doubt whether improvement reflected what we properly call learning. What do you think?

When Thorndike performed this experiment around the beginning of this century, nothing at all was known about the neuro-physical foundation of learning. Relatively little more is known today, but the kind of motor skill explored in Game 6.2 is better understood. It is principally the work of the cerebellum (see Chapter 2).

II

E. L. Thorndike was one of the founders of that vast excrescence on psychology called learning theory. For sixty years, psychologists focused their attention on the accumulation of data from experiments with animals out of which they distilled an elaborate and highly speculative brew. Rats lead the list of experimental animals, but mice, guinea pigs and other rodents, primates from monkeys to apes, dogs, cats, pigeons and goldfish have played their roles by devoting their boring lives to science. The technique was to use a stimulus to produce a response out of which it was possible to mould a new condition, in other words, a conditioned response. The behaviourists are also interested in the extinction of a conditioned response, using the same techniques they employed to obtain it. Pavlov's original experiments taught dogs to salivate at the sound of a bell rather than at the appearance of food. His work was criticized because animals in the wild have a chance to respond so as to change the stimulus; that is, they can eat the food. At Harvard University, B. F. Skinner began a study of animals kept in boxes designed so that they could reward themselves with food pellets for correct responses. Thus, learning theory moved from the technique known as classical conditioning to that known as operant conditioning, also called instrumental learning.

You can observe the effects of your classical conditioning in the things that make you feel close to tears. Do you cry, for example, when a pet animal dies during a film? Obviously, not everyone does, but your response has been learned and is very hard to suppress. Or if you have stopped smoking, do you ever feel a strong craving at some particular time, say at the end of a long or a heavy meal (but see the end of this chapter on addiction). The chances are that this feeling, too, is a reflection of classical conditioning that has been largely, though not entirely, extinguished.

As to operant conditioning, Skinner maintains that it goes on being the mode of all learning throughout life. We learn to buy fashionable clothes, for example, not only because of advertising, but also because we have been conditioned to respond with feelings of comfort and discomfort to the social norms displayed by others.

Conditioning experiments provide results which are highly quantifiable. Behaviourism claimed to be the first experimental psychology capable of producing objective, statistically-useful scientific data about learning. In order to make the claim, it was necessary to jettison old-fashioned subjective concepts such as consciousness, memory and emotion which could not be tested within the parameters fixed by the alleged unit of behaviour: stimulus-response. Behaviourism is the theoretical framework which gave birth to learning theory.

There is certainly much to be learned about ourselves by analogy with animal behaviour in conditioning experiments, especially those using instrumental learning techniques.

Thus, for an infant, crying is an instrument to assuage hunger. Food is a response which reinforces the usefulness of crying, and the satisfied infant stops crying. Note that the mother uses food as a stimulus to produce silence. Having learned that crying brings food, the infant generalizes the discovery: he cries when he wants company. If he cries at two o' clock in the morning and his parents sensibly refuse to pick him up, that part of the crying instrument meant to bring company during the night is extinguished. The infant learns that he may cry to satisfy 'real' needs; that is, those recognized as real by his parents. In other words, he learns to discriminate and to apply the crying instrument appropriately.

As with all behaviourist evidence, there tends to be contradictory evidence. Thus, tests have also shown that babies whose parents always pick them up cry less at one year old than those who have not been picked up, and yet other tests reveal that the best treatment is inconsistency, a blessed finding for most parents, surely! These contradictions suggest that the experiments themselves are faulty – a common phenomenon in science.

The behaviourist approach to learning reveals the relationship between facets of behaviour, but it does not help us to understand another class of questions. Why, for example, does the infant cry to attract attention? How does he know that a loud, continuous noise is likely to bring help? If he is hungry, presumably he needs food to form energy. It could be argued that silence would at least conserve the energy of a hungry baby.

Or consider the other side of the equation. The mother responds to crying because the noise is felicitously calculated to drive her crazy. The infant smiles, and the smile too has a potent effect on the mother. Why? How did the infant acquire smile behaviour in the first place? By observing the mother? Because questions of origin and meaning lie outside the stimulus-response behaviour unit, behaviourists have usually set them aside as worthless.

As a result of their single-minded concentration on the

stimulus-response unit, some behaviourists found themselves in another quandary. Language is a very nearly universal human behaviour. Many people believe, however, that it is exclusively human. Eating, sleeping, fornicating, even the use of tools, are activities that humans share with many other animal species, but these other species cannot talk. The stimulus-response approach can be brought to bear on language, but not by using animal experiments. More important, if language is not a behaviour that humans share with other animals, then it is at least possible that the human brain grows in a different way because humans inherit different genes, in which case language is in some part not a learned behaviour at all.

The behaviourists deny that humans alone can use language. Their insistence – and their influence on bodies that give money to research – has provided several apes and chimpanzees and a number of scientists with a happy if unfruitful relationship, especially in the United States. People first tried to teach apes to speak a century ago. About 1905, a few primate specialists realized that apes would not mimic what they heard, but that they do try to mimic what they see. After World War II, this fact was given practical effect. B. T. and R. A. Gardner trained a chimpanzee named Washoe in the use of a simplified version of American sign language, itself a modification of the hand signals used by the deaf-and-dumb. Using operational conditioning methods, the Gardners taught their charge some eighty-five signs in three years. Washoe had apparently also invented some of her own, for example, a sign for *bib*. In that way she seemed to have acquired one of the essential attributes of language, the ability to create new words or word groups to fit new situations. Several other experimenters have varied the Gardners' techniques, and all of them have reported some success. It began to look as though other animals could learn a language even though it might be minimal.

More recently, doubts have arisen. For example, the Gardners had simplified or reduced Washoe's answers to certain phrases. 'You me you out me' was taken by them to mean 'you me'. They reasoned that the repetitions were not significant and that the content, 'you me', was what counted for Washoe as well as for themselves. But is that true? Three-year-old children tend to prune words from their meaningful sentences, not to add unnecessary ones. 'Car' can mean either, 'I want to go for a ride in the car,' or 'That is a car,' or even 'Where is my car?', depending on the context. Unlike Washoe, young children appear to use fewer words to carry more weight.

An American psychologist, Herbert S. Terrace, is one of the latest experimenters in this field. He has written an unusually honest book called *Nim*, the name he gave to his chimpanzee. In all the studies, gestures made by the trained chimpanzees were filmed. Terrace pointed out that when outside observers have tried to 'read' the filmed talk, they have often failed. He hoped to avoid this problem by employing several teachers who had to agree that Nim had used a sign before he was credited with having learned it. Like Washoe and other primates, Nim learned many signs and used them freely with his teachers, but Terrace was not convinced that Nim understood that there were grammatical relationships, for example, between 'eat' and 'me'. Outside rigid two- or at best three-word limits, furthermore, Nim could not make sentences. He showed none of the insistence upon language, the incessant questioning and chattering of a three-year-old child. Beyond a small number of instinctual grunts, the primates certainly do not develop language as a common means of exchange with their own kind. Neither do they 'talk' to other trained primates, nor do they try to teach signs. At best, the behaviourist case for denying human uniqueness in language use remains unproven.

Meanwhile, the American professor of linguistics, Noam Chomsky, launched a direct attack on the behaviourist interpretation of language learning as a complex conditioned response. Chomsky pointed out that if a child learned solely by imitation and reward, there seemed to be no reason for the common aspects of language development. Why say 'goed' instead of 'went', 'doed' for 'did', 'sheeps' or 'you naughty are'?. Yet each of these formal mistakes makes sense if you assume that in addition to imitating sounds, the importance of which can hardly be denied, each child brings something else to bear on his need to express himself. The words 'goed' and 'doed' fit the most common method of making an English past tense: adding '-ed' to make, for instance, wanted, placed, loved. Went and did are irregular verbs. Similarly, 'sheeps' obeys the common rule for making plurals. Most interesting of all is 'you naughty are'. The meaning is perfectly clear. The child's error lies in having arranged the words in the order of their importance, a common feature of many English sentences. For example: 'Climb up here.' 'Here, climb up.' 'Up here, climb!' The child has acquired the ability not just to imitate but to imitate creatively using the acceptable rules of grammar long before he has been taught them. Chomsky suggested that this is possible because the child inherits rules of grammar – not the rules of *English* grammar, of course, but universal rules applicable to all languages. They come with human brain structure.

You can see what a hash this makes of traditional stimulus-response learning theory. If parts of our language capacity are inherited, then what about other kinds of behaviour? And not just human behaviour. Slowly, instincts and emotions, followed by motivations and consciousness, began to creep back into psychology. Then the whole process speeded up because improved laboratory technology made it possible to examine the activity of groups of neurons when a behaviour was being learned. As we have seen, the hippocampus appears to play a role in the consolidation of long-term memory, particularly with respect to spatial relationships. Some neurons involved in vision appear to have to learn how to see (see Chapter 8). In other words, there is growing neurophysiological support for the belief that in addition to experience, learning could not take place without at least a bent or capacity.

Neurophysiology actually goes a step further in undermining classical learning theory. It calls into question the unitary nature of a stimulus and a response. For example, a rat responds to a pellet of food dropped into a cup. What he sees and hears is not food but a series of lines, curves and sound frequencies. He has previously learned to associate them with a smell, let us say, and the smell is in turn associated with the quality 'edible'. A whole series of neurons and neuronal networks appears to be associated. Yet each neuron signals after a separate stimulus. Any part of the system could drop out, and the response might or might not be changed. In any case, the apparent unity of a stimulus is illusory. Similarly, the unitary response can be seen as a whole sequence of muscular adjustments requiring complex nervous control. As has been the case with the atom, an indivisible unit has shattered into many smaller events. Perhaps this is one reason for the contradictory results often produced by behavioural experiments.

III

Chomsky called the built-in universal rules of grammar 'deep structures'. There is no physiological evidence for the existence of deep structures. Nor is there much physiological evidence for memory. Yet no one denies that memory exists. In support of Chomsky's theory, consider these two sentences:

> Mother is cooking.
> Supper is cooking.

The surface grammatical structure is the same: noun, auxilliary verb, verb (or: noun, verb, participle). Indeed, but for the nouns, the two sentences are identical. But 'mother' is active and 'supper' is passive. How do I know that?

Game 6.3: When did you last analyse a sentence? It used to be called parsing. I can remember my fourth-grade teacher drawing on the blackboard diagrams like Figure 6.1.

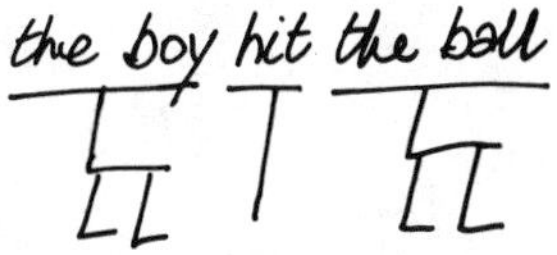

Fig. 6.1

Here is another kind of parsing based on Chomskian rules of phrase structure. Each rule is expressed in symbols and in ordinary English. The sentence being parsed is again: The boy hit the ball.

Rules	*Strings (of symbols)*
1 S → NP + VP	S
Rewrite sentence as noun phrase plus verb phrase.	NP + VP
2 VP → Verb + NP	NP + Verb + NP
Rewrite verb phrase as verb plus noun phrase.	
3 NP → { NPsing, NPpl }	NPsing + Verb + NP
Rewrite noun phrase as noun phrase singular or noun phrase plural.	
Rule 3 applies a second time.	NPsing + Verb + NPsing
4 NPsing → T + N + Ø	T + N + Ø + Verb + NPsing
Rewrite noun phrase singular as article (T) plus noun (N) with no inflection (Ø).	
Rule 4 applies a second time.	T + N + Ø + Verb + T + N + Ø
5 NPpl → T + N + 's	Rule 5 does not apply.
Rewrite noun phrase in plural as article plus noun plus 's inflection.	

6	T → *the, a* Substitute word for article symbol (i.e., T).	*the* + N + Ø + Verb + T + N + Ø
	Rule 6 applies a second time.	*the* + N + Ø + Verb + *the* + N + Ø
7	N → *boy, ball*, etc. Substitute some word for noun symbol.	*the* + *boy* + Ø + Verb + *the* + N + Ø
	Rule 7 applies a second time.	*the* + *boy* + Ø + Verb + *the* + *ball* + Ø
8	Verb → Aux + V Rewrite Verb as Auxilliary plus V.	*the* + *boy* + Ø + Aux + V + *the* + *ball* + Ø
9	V → *hit, take, walk,* *read*, etc. Substitute word for verb symbol (V).	*the* + *boy* + Ø + Aux + *hit* + *the* + *ball* + Ø
10	Aux → C(M) (have + en) (ne + ing) Rewrite auxilliary for tense (obligatory) and as modal, perfective or progressive (all optional).	*the* + *boy* + Ø + C + *hit* + *the* + *ball* + Ø
11	M → *will, can, may,* *shall, must* Substitute word for modal symbol.	Rule 11 does not apply. String unchanged.

12	C → ⎰ 's in the context
	     NPsing
	   O in other
	      context
	   past in any
	      context ⎱
	Rewrite tense as inflection
	with noun phrase in
	singular, or as no inflection
	in other contexts,
	or as past in any context.
		the + *boy* + Ø + past + *hit*
		+ *the* + *ball* + Ø

The first eleven rules are properly called phrase-structure rules. The twelfth offers a choice of three alternatives each of which could transform the symbols into a completed sentence. In this instance, only the third is possible. Make up your own sentence and use this technique to analyse it. Does the analysis suggest to you anything about the nature of a universal grammar?

This exercise indicates how Chomsky developed what he called the transformational grammar in which deep structure embodied in symbols related to each other by phrase-structure rules are converted into surface structure; that is, the sentences we speak or write. By their nature, the phrase-structure rules should be applicable to any language.

Chomsky has modified his already complicated system to meet criticism of the way it works as a logical system of symbols. (Mathematics is also the study of logical systems of symbols, one of which is called arithmetic.) Yet as I said, there is no concrete evidence for the existence of deep structures. Nevertheless, the logical foundations of grammar formed in some such way have provided a tool for development of computers that talk. These machines have been programmed, using rules of transformational grammar, to answer questions and to distinguish rational from irrational conversational gambits.

In the following recorded conversation between a human and a computer, the human voice is in italics.

Men are all alike.
In what way
They're always bugging us about something or other.
Can you think of a specific example
Well, my boyfriend made me come here.
Your boyfriend made you come here
He says I'm depressed most of the time.
I am sorry to hear you are depressed
It's true. I am unhappy.
Do you think coming here will help you not to be unhappy
I need some help, that much seems certain.

What would it mean to you if you got some help
Perhaps I could learn to get along with my mother.
Tell me more about your family
My mother takes care of me.
Who else in your family takes care of you
My father.
Your father
You are like my father in some ways.
What resemblance do you see
You are not very aggressive but I think you don't want me to notice that.
What makes you think I am not very aggressive
You don't argue with me.
Why do you think I don't argue with you
You are afraid of me.
Does it please you to believe I am afraid of you
My father is afraid of everybody.
What else comes to mind when you think of your father
Bullies.
Does that have anything to do with the fact that your boyfriend made you come here

Note how the computer copes with a logical non-sequitur; for example, the human reply: 'My father is afraid of everybody'. Do you think the computer 'understands' what it has said? Is there any way of testing the computer to determine whether its understanding is like human understanding?

Chomsky's deep structures are an example of the models in the brain which I mentioned in the chapter on memory. Though there is no proof that deep structures exist, science is always looking for the simplest explanation of the data. Does it not seem simpler to believe in the presence of certain formal relationships emerging out of nervous structure than it would be to instill the magnificent originality of language by a crescendo of stimulus-response learning? But if deep structures exist, why can they not be located? As we have seen, the evidence is against such localization. Again, it seems simpler to theorize that such models are scattered. They are filed in the brain by some system which is still unrecognized. There is circumstantial evidence to support this hypothesis.

Game 6.4: Sound the letters: f, v. Now, form: p, b. Sound each of the consonants without a vowel sound.

Each letter requires both a puff of air and a set of the lips and teeth, but the first two letters vary whereas the second pair are the same. Anyone who can read has made each adjustment automatically, and it is reasonable to assume that because different muscles are required to make them, different brain areas are also involved. The throat and lip regions are under the control of separate motor centres, the left parieto-temporal speech centre regulates actual sound, and the left temporal lobe language comprehension centre is in charge of understanding the instructions. Perhaps such distribution is evidence that language data are scattered throughout the cortex.

I tie a knot in a handkerchief to remind myself of something; a purely physical act involving an intrinsically meaningless symbol to recall something meaningful. Mnemonics and the 'times' tables are devices to 'tie knots in the activities of man's brain', A. R. Luria has written, to link together the different brain centres involved. Perhaps the most striking piece of circumstantial evidence supporting the idea of deep structures is the not-infrequent case of the left-hemisphere-damaged adult who can still write – such as Luria's patient who kept his own journal (see Chapter 2). Luria believes that his ability reflects the 'conversion of writing ... from a process requiring precise acoustic analysis into a motor automatism', a role that may be played by the cerebellum. In other words, when you learn to write, the learning takes place not only in the language-regulating centres but also in the motor centres of the cortex and in the cerebellum. Perhaps learning links together in-built models, such as deep structures, with acquired motor and phonetic skills.

There is one specialized form of learning that might hold a clue: addiction. Do you smoke, or did you ever smoke? Most of us still fall into one category or the other. Think for a minute about what it is that causes you to reach for the next cigarette. How do you feel when you reach? If you will also try to recall how you once managed without cigarettes, or perhaps, if you are lucky, how you can manage without whereas once you could not – if you can bring to mind both conditions simultaneously, you will appreciate that smoking is a kind of learning. So is addiction to alcohol, heroin or any other drug.

In part at least, addiction reflects the physio-chemical changes in neurons caused by the drugs. Morphine is both the most effective pain-killer and one of the most addictive drugs. Much research has been devoted to understanding its mechanism of action in neurons. As long ago as 1900, the German bacteriologist, Paul Ehrlich, suggested that drugs work by linking up with a specialized molecule on the cell membrane, a sort of lock-and-key arrangement which opens the cell to the new drug molecule. Although the lock-and-key analogy is far too simple, the receptor on the cell membrane is now an established part of biochemical doctrine because there is much evidence that such molecules do exist. If a drug like morphine can exert a beneficial effect, therefore, a receptor for it must exist on some neurons. But a receptor could not have evolved in the cell membrane on the off chance that a drug called morphine would be extracted from the opium poppy by a German chemist named Sertürner in 1803. The receptor must have evolved because there is a natural pain-killer that uses it. (It might be argued with equal force that the pain-killer evolved because the receptor for it existed. From our standpoint, priority is irrelevant.) In any case, a natural pain-killer would be unlikely to cause addiction. In 1975, building on the work of earlier researchers, Dr John Hughes and his associates at the University of Aberdeen isolated such a natural pain-killer. They named it enkephalin. Enkephalin is not yet accepted as a drug, but there are several closely related natural chemicals and the search goes on for a non-addictive pain-killer embodying an enkephalin-like molecule. Because pain is a complex sensation involving the cerebral cortex as well as mid-brain centres such as the thalamus (see Chapter 7), addiction could involve neurons in one location, and pain control those in another. The enkephalin story does seem to establish the fact, however, that there is a distinction between the addictive and the pain-killing activities of morphine.

Enkephalin, or one of its related substances, may act like any other chemical inhibitory transmitter of a neuronal signal. It seems to inhibit the firing of a post-synaptic neuron, slowing or stopping pain sensations. Morphine makes pain bearable, but it does not actually stop it. The drug may displace enkephalin from the receptor molecule for it, at the same time causing some other change to take place either in the same neuron or in some other cell. To kill pain, therefore, more of the drug is needed – one of the symptoms of addiction.

To see the connection I am proposing between addiction and learning, you need only think back to the supposed chemical nature of long-term memory. The 'addicted neuron' is chemically-different from the normal neuron. What is more, addiction may occur in different parts of the brain – in the case of morphine, in the cortex and the thalamus. Is this diffusion merely an analogy to the learning process, or is there some real similarity between addiction and learning?

Stimulus-response learning theory grew up before biochemistry. Today the study of learning behaviour concentrates on the physical nature of memory, on the development of the human infant, and on sensation because it is the origin of all experience. Conditioning experiments may still be useful tools in all three areas of research.

7   Sensation I: Touch, Taste, Balance and Hearing

I

Game 7.1: Unless you have a windowless room available, this game is best played at night. Exclude as much light as possible. You will need either two flashlights or two lamps with the same wattage bulbs. Turn on one light source and let your eyes adjust. About 30 seconds will do. Then turn on the second light. You have now doubled the light in the room. Does the room seem to you to be twice as light, half again as light, or does it seem to have about the same degree of lightness? The chances are that your answer will fall between the same and half again as much.

Doubling the light usually produces an impression that the brightness has increased by about a quarter. If you turn on a third light of the same size, the average impression will be that brightness has increased by roughly 44 per cent over the first light – still less than half although the light source has tripled. The increment between the second and the third light is also smaller than between the first and second.

Although Game 7.1 uses vision, and this chapter is devoted to the other senses, it illustrates perhaps the earliest strictly psychological law ever formulated. In 1854 Ernst Heinrich Weber stated that the stronger the original stimulus, the larger the increment required to be noticeable. A match lit in a dark room is very noticeable, but in a brightly-lit room it can hardly be seen. However, if a mild electric shock is followed by a shock from double the current, the increment may seem much more than twice as much – an experiment that I strongly urge you NOT TO TRY.

At the extremes Weber's law does not hold. For example, a very small decrease in a painfully-loud noise may be easily noticed. A lighted cigarette will shine out brightly on a dark night. These two examples introduce a new psychological phenomenon, the just-noticeable-difference or j.n.d.

Game 7.2: Make several coloured pieces of paper of about the same size, say two inches square. Each piece should be a single colour: red, orange, yellow, green, blue, purple. Ask a friend to sit so that he can see the colours easily in a good light. Ask him to speak or hold up his hand when he sees blue. Show him the pieces of paper as quickly as you can with blue towards the end or in the middle. Your subject may call green or purple blue, but he will almost never mistake red, yellow or orange for blue.

Game 7.3: While your friend is still sitting comfortably, ask him to tell you as soon as he hears the sound from your radio. You will have pretuned the radio to a strong station and turned it on with the volume right down so that there is no sound at all. After instructing your subject, shield your hand with your body or a piece of furniture so that he cannot see it move. Turn the dial very slowly until your friend stops you. Mark the point reached with a soft pencil. Turn the radio down again. Repeat the test five times. How close has your subject come to the original mark? The average of the five marks is his j.n.d. for sound in the conditions (noise and other distractions) applying during the game.

In 1860 another German experimental psychologist, G. T. Fechner, described the just-noticeable-difference as the subjective magnitude of a sensation measured by the logarithm of the physical magnitude of its stimulus. Some examples of this are:

A tone of 2000 cycles per second can be heard when the movement of air particles against the eardrum is smaller than the diameter of a molecule.

One part of a gas, mercaptan, can be detected in 50 million parts of air.

If the senses were any more sensitive, they would respond to random molecular movements. There is already 'noise' in the nervous system caused by the random firing of neurons. If it were increased by excessive sensitivity, a subjective impression of chaos would ensue. Indeed, it is possible that some works of art reflect just such extreme sensitivity on the part of the artist. One thinks, for example, of the later paintings of Van Gogh.

The senses depend on sensory apparatus which has three anatomical parts. The first part, the receptor, may be a single specialized neuron, as in the sense of touch, or a highly-elaborate combination of specialized neurons arranged in a complex organ, such as the ear. The second part of the apparatus is a nervous connection to the central nervous system. Touch connects by a single neuron to the spinal cord where it can effect a reflex action by means of only two connections. Just such a physiological connection is the machinery you use when you jerk your finger away from a flame. The retina of the eye is also linked by only two connections to the visual cortex. Touch sensations carried to the brain, however, require as many as four connections. Finally, there is a discrete brain centre receiving the message from a sense organ. Unlike memory traces, brain neurons signalling the sensory inputs are often precisely identified. Many have already been described in Chapter 2.

Vernon Mountcastle, the American neurophysiologist, has written that the sense organs answer six questions:

1   Has anything happened, is anything there or is the sensation merely 'noise' in the system?
2   What is it?
3   How much of it is there?
4   Is this stimulus stronger than some other occurring at the same time or just previously? (J.n.d. is a special aspect of this question).
5   Where is it?
6   Is the stimulus changing in space or time?

The rest of this chapter is organized by sensation. Classically, there are five senses, but we shall explore eight: taste and smell, touch (including pressure and temperature), pain, proprioception, balance, hearing and seeing, the last being the subject of Chapter 8.

II

Taste, smell and touch are sometimes called the minor senses. By contrast, hearing and seeing are major senses. Of course this is judging from the human standpoint. If one measures the amount of cortex devoted to the respective senses, the so-called minor senses are major in other animals. Humans can survive without a sense of taste (ageusia), and many people are wholly or partly anosmic, that is, they have an impaired sense of smell. Touch is vitally important, but there are rare individuals lacking at least a sense of pain. Nevertheless, the minor senses grow in significance when there is an impairment of hearing or seeing, and in the absence of major senses, taste, smell and touch remain. Helen Keller was an American girl born deaf and blind. By the most Herculean effort, she learned to speak, read and write. This is a small excerpt from her account of her teacher's arrival and of an early teaching experience:

> I guessed from my mother's signs and from hurrying to and fro in the house that something unusual was about to happen, so I went to the door and waited on the steps. The afternoon sun penetrated the mass of honeysuckle that covered the porch, and fell on my upturned face. My fingers lingered almost unconsciously on the familiar leaves and blossoms which had just come forth to greet the sweet southern spring. I did not know what the future held of marvel or surprise for me.... We walked down the path to the well-house, attracted by the fragrance of the honeysuckle with which it was covered. Someone was drawing water and my teacher held my hand under the spout. As the cold stream gushed over one hand....

Taste and smell are separate senses. Each has its own sense organ and nervous connections to different brain regions. They influence each other but largely by association of sensations in the cortex. Everyone knows that a nasty smell affects our perception of taste. Both taste and smell are chemical senses: they depend on the binding of molecules in the air or in food and drink by receptors on specialized neurons.

The organs of taste, the taste buds, are in the back of the mouth and on the tongue. Taste depends on four classes of sensation: sour, salt, bitter and sweet. The taste buds are groups of twenty or thirty specialized neurons which respond to a minimum of two and perhaps to all four taste classes. They are concentrated at the tip of the tongue, which is more sensitive to sweet tastes; the edges of the tongue, which are most sensitive to sour and salt; and the root, sensitive to bitterness.

Game 7.4: You can test at least the first two of these localizations. Use a pinch of sugar, a pinch of salt and a small measure of vinegar. Try placing very small amounts of each substance first on the tip of the tongue and then in the cheek so that it will come into contact with the side of the tongue. Be sure to rinse your mouth with cool water after each tasting.

With age, taste acuity declines. It is thought that this represents nothing more sinister than the frictional wearing away of the nerve endings in the taste buds. A blow to the head can cause loss of taste sensation, but this is usually temporary. No one knows quite what happens because there is no single primary taste area in the brain analogous, for example, to the olfactory bulb, the forward portion of the mid-brain out of which the cortex has evolved.

Game 7.5: The sensitivity of your nose to smells can be demonstrated, but you must take care. Do *not* attempt this experiment if the gas burner on your stove lights auto-

matically from a pilot light. Stand erect and facing the gas
stove, press against it. Turn the gas burner directly below
your face full on and turn it off again as quickly as you
can. Do not leave it on, but make the on-off movement
continuous. You should smell gas almost as quickly as you
complete the movement.

The olfactory nerves in the nose are concentrated in an area
about the size of a fingernail in the roof of each nostril.
Each neuron is specialized for one class of smell, such as
acrid or smoky. Man-made smells, like bread baking, are
probably learned from the association of smell classes in
the cortex.

The olfactory neurons are linked to the olfactory bulb
at the front of the mid-brain. In non-human animals the
olfactory bulb is much larger in relation to brain size, and
their visual and aural centres are proportionally smaller.
Seeing and hearing permit subtler and more discriminatory
sensations than does smell, and it is possible that we are
cleverer than other animals simply because we are better
informed.

III

It takes time for a sensation to move from the sense organ
to the brain. If the time required is more than one millisecond (msec: 0.001 of a second), touch sensations from
different parts of your body are localized at the spot nearest
the brain.

Game 7.6: Touch your index finger tips together lightly and
rapidly. Most people report an equal sensation from both
fingertips.

Now, touch one index finger tip lightly and quickly
against a lip. In this case though the finger tip and the lip
are both rich in touch-sensing neurons, the sensation will
probably come from the lip. It takes a little more than one

msec longer for a message to reach the brain from the fingertip than from the lip. Finally, touch your index finger lightly and rapidly against your ankle bone or your big toe. Where do you feel the sensation this time? Most people will reply, from the fingertip. It takes just over one msec longer for a message to reach the brain from the ankle or toe than it does from the finger tip.

Like the neurons in other sense organs, the touch sensors display a quality called adaptation. They signal when the stimulus first appears, but if it remains unvarying, the sensing neurons stop signalling. The physio-chemical reason for this can be made clear in the case of the light-sensitive rod and cone cells of the eye (Chapter 8), but the touch sensors are less well understood. Adaptation is not the same as the refractory period (see Chapter 2) during which the neuron is unable to signal because it is recovering from the previous signal. Nor is it the same as adaptability, a quality of intelligence (see Chapter 4). Adaptation is excellent evidence that what counts for the organism is newness rather than sameness. Adaptation to a stimulus leaves the sensory apparatus open to the latest thing.

Game 7.7: You can demonstrate adaptation of the touch sensors with two small circles of cardboard. One should be about ½ in. in diameter and the other about 2 in. You will also need a watch with a second hand and a co-operative friend. Ask your friend to lie face down with the back bare. Lay one cardboard circle on the back and time the period until your friend reports that the sensation from it has stopped. Do the same with the second piece of cardboard. Now, repeat the test, applying a light pressure from your finger tips against each cardboard circle. You should find that the lighter touch (that is, before you pressed) and the larger surface show the fastest adaptation.

In addition to localization and adaptation, the touch sensors display a third characteristic: they each have an excitatory region surrounded by an inhibitory region. A similar phenomenon is found in the visual system. In the case of touch the exact neuronal machinery underlying the phenomenon is not clear, but you can demonstrate its reality.

Game 7.8: You need two sharply-pointed objects, such as tooth picks or stiff broom bristles. Do *not* use knives because it is necessary to apply pressure against the skin during the experiment. It will also work best if a friend controls the stimuli though you can do it yourself.

First, press with one point against the skin of your palm. Note how the sensation comes from a well-defined circular region. Now, press in the same spot with the two points together. You should still feel only one point. Continue to press the palm with two points applying pressure firmly, releasing it and reapplying after a brief delay, but each time you reapply pressure, move the points a little further apart. Pay close attention to what you feel. At first you should still feel only one point. Then just as you sense two points, you should discover that instead, both sensations fade, and the pressure at both points seems to be reduced. It is important that you maintain the same pressure at each application of the two points, of course. When you next move them a bit further apart, you will again feel two distinct points.

What has happened to you can be described with the help of Figure 7.1.

Game 7.8 depends on pressure and Game 7.6 on fine touch. These forms of touch stimulate single neurons, the specialized dendrites of which are encapsulated in several concentric skin layers forming corpuscles. They are called Pacinian corpuscles, after the Italian anatomist who described them. There are two other kinds of touch sensors, however. Groups of unencapsulated neurons respond to rough touch, such as stretching. Single more or less isolated neurons sense temperature and probably pain. Both physiologically and subjectively these three aspects of touch are

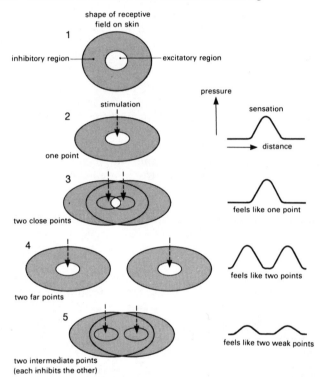

Fig. 7.1: Inhibitory interactions on the skin

continuous. Pressure from the point of a toothpick begins as touch and involves stretching. Both pressure and temperature may become painful. This characteristic arises both because of the behaviour of the specialized neurons which respond over a range of stimulus activity and from the manner in which the touch sensations reach the brain.

Touch neurons from each skin area form nerve trunks, often visible to the naked eye. Each trunk runs to the spinal cord at the appropriate level; that is, arms in the upper part of the back, legs at the bottom. In the spinal cord the sensing neurons synapse with interneurons. These may synapse in turn with a neuron running back to a muscle in the area from which the sensation originated thus forming the basis of a reflex action. The same interneuron may also synapse with a neuron running to the brain. In either case the group of sensations from a skin area are signalled together. In the cord and the specialized sensory regions of the brain, moreover, the sensations from a skin area travel in relation to signals from other areas so that together they form an homunculus or map of the body. Sensations of touch that reach the brain are mixtures of touch, pressure and temperature from each skin area, and they are localized. The colliculi, on the hind-brain, and the sensory cortex are the primary areas of touch sensation.

You are probably aware that some parts of your body are more sensitive than others. There are many more neurons sensing touch in the palm than in the back. The highest concentrations are in the big toes and the soles of the feet. In both sexes the breasts are more sensitive than the palms. The first (index) finger tip is more sensitive than the other three fingers or the thumb.

Game 7.9: With light touches, you can easily demonstrate the differences in sensitivity over your body and construct your own subjective diagram to compare with the generalized charts in Figures 7.2a and b. Figure 7.2a shows pressure thresholds for women; that is, the level of pressure to which the brain first responds. Figure 7.2b charting pressure thresholds for men is similar, but the average thresholds are a little higher.

In other words women are, on the whole, more sensitive to pressure than men. It is arguable, however, whether women are also subjectively less capable of bearing pain. Childbirth is considered to be the most painful natural process, but the fixing of objective standards to judge pain is notoriously difficult.

Pain is a separate sense only to the degree that pain sensation depends in part on a separate sensory neuron, though even

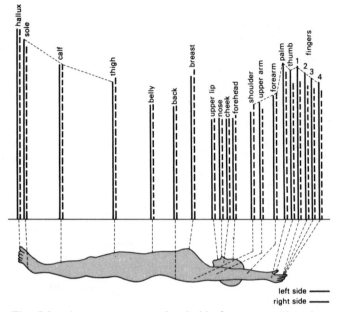

left side ———
right side ———

Fig. 7.2a: Average pressure thresholds for women (based on S. Weinstein in D. R. Kenshalo [ed.], *The Skin Senses*, Charles C. Thomas, 1968)

this sensor is also responsible for temperature. It seems probable that pressure sensors also convey pain sensations and, indeed, the rough touch receptors may do so with suitable provocation.

Game 7.10: Ask a friend to grasp your forearm firmly with both hands and to twist them in the opposite directions. You will soon want him to stop. Presumably this rough touch is stimulating the complexes of unencapsulated neuron endings in the skin of your forearm.

Thus we approach what has been called appropriately, 'the puzzle of pain'. There is no single pain receptor, no pain pathway to the brain and no brain centre exclusively devoted to pain. Like touch, pain sensitivity varies on different parts

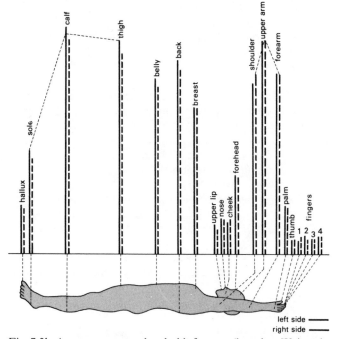

Fig. 7.2b: Average pressure thresholds for men (based on Weinstein in Kenshalo, *The Skin Senses*)

of the body. The back of the knee, the neck and the elbow bend are most sensitive whereas the sole of the foot and the tip of the nose – both regions high in touch receptors – are least sensitive.

The survival value of pain is obvious. Yet of all the sensations, pain may be most affected by emotion, attention and other seemingly extraneous factors. We are brought up to believe, for example, that little boys don't cry, but little girls may. Fakirs and saints have withstood laceration, burning and other tortures which would reduce most of us to a quaking jelly. Soldiers in the midst of battle suffer wounds which they do not seem to notice until the danger has passed. Evidently the cerebral cortex plays a major role in regulating pain sensation.

There is no way to measure your pain threshold, but it is possible to determine whether it is relatively high or low and to compare your own threshold to that of others.

Game 7.11: Answer the following question by scoring yourself between the extremes on a scale measured from 1 (greatest resistance to pain or high pain threshold) to 5 (least resistance or lowest threshold).

1   Do you consider yourself to be:
    Stoical and serious-minded? (1)
    Halfway between? (3)
    Easy-going and comfort-seeking? (5)
2   Can you carry hot plates to the table bare-handed?
    Always (1)
    Depends (3)
    Never (5)
3   Do you fear an injection administered by a doctor, dentist or nurse?
    Not at all (1)
    Quite a lot (3)
    Very much (5)
4   Do you have a local anesthetic when a dentist drills a tooth?
    Never (1)
    Sometimes (3)
    Always (5)
5   Do you carefully protect a finger which has received a minor cut?
    Never (1)
    Sometimes (3)
    Always (5)
6   What would you do if you twisted your ankle on stepping off a curb?
    Try to walk on limping as little as possible (1)
    Hop (3)
    Sit down where you are and wait for help (5)

7 What would your attitude be if you needed major surgery?

Accept it as necessary (1)

Agree, but not without hesitation (3)

Seek alternative forms of treatment (5)

8 If you have a severe headache or arthritic pain, do you:

Remain silent? (1)

Put on a brave front in public? (3)

Moan despairingly and go to bed? (5)

Add up your score. The higher it is, the lower your pain threshold appears to be.

There is still no simple, convincing explanation of pain. The most useful theory was proposed in the late 1960s by Patrick Wall and Ronald Melzack, British and Canadian neurophysiologists respectively. It is called the gate theory because it depends upon the existence within the spinal cord of a neuronal gate. If the gate is open, pain signals reach the brain; if it is closed, they cannot.

The putative gate consists of two sorts of sensory neurons. We have seen in Chapter 2 that large, myelinated axons conduct much faster than small unmyelinated axons. The larger neurons also respond to less stimulation than the small neurons. In the case of pain, both kinds of neurons conduct signals from the different touch receptors, and the large neurons have a lower threshold than the small ones. Large neurons, therefore, deliver pain signals to the spinal cord first. According to the theory, one of the interneurons they stimulate is inhibitory, preventing signals from going up to the brain but leaving any reflex response unimpaired. Thus, the large, fast neuron closes the gate. The small, slow neuron, on the other hand, stimulates inhibitory interneurons inhibiting signals from the large neurons, as in Figure 7.3. The slow signal delivered by the small neuron opens the gate. Learning and attention play a role because signals from the cortex descend the spinal cord and either increase the inhibition of messages to the brain or reduce inhibition further opening the gate.

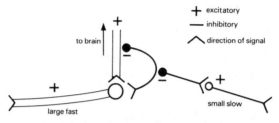

Fig. 7.3: Arrangement of neurons in the gate

No physical evidence of a gate has yet been unequivocally demonstrated. In medicine however, one test of a theory is: does treatment based on it help the patient? According to the gate theory, to reduce pain the gate must be kept closed. To close the gate, it is necessary to stimulate the low-threshold, large neurons but not the high-threshold, small neurons. It is possible to deliver low threshold stimuli by means of a weak electrical current, and there have been some successes in treating pain by this method. At first the stimulus came from electrodes on the skin. If the gate is in the spinal cord, however, it seemed a good idea to implant small radio receivers near the cord which would emit a mild current on the order of a transmitter carried either by the patient or by the doctor. In early trials the efficacy of this surgical procedure seemed doubtful, but towards the end of the 1970s new tests using carefully-selected patients have had better results. Implants in the brain itself have also been tried. They have been placed near the thalamus, the centre which acts as a relay station both for incoming touch sensations and for outgoing movement orders. They have been moderately successful, but probably not because they affect the theoretical gate. Brain implants are thought to stimulate neurons to synthesize the natural pain-killer, enkephalin (see Chapter 6). Evidence from clinical trials of all these techniques is still inconclusive.

The mild electric current could also act as what is commonly called a counter-irritant, like pushing your finger against your upper lip to stop a sneeze. Counter-irritation might well utilize a gating mechanism.

Acupuncture has been used to induce anesthesia only since the Communist Revolution in China, though it is of course an ancient technique for the treatment of disease. It is thought that at certain acupuncture points the needle stimulates large, low-threshold sensory neurons closing the putative gate. There are other possible explanations. An element of suggestion may be involved when acupuncture controls pain. The Chinese will not use it for anesthesia if the patient wishes to have chemical anesthesia, or if he doubts the efficacy of acupuncture. It is not used during childbirth or to anesthetize small children. On the other hand, there is some biochemical evidence that the needles cause neurons to release enkephalin or one of the related chemicals. The needles can be very painful themselves, though, and acupuncturists use this pain as one indication that the treatment has gone on long enough. In any case though it is still not scientifically well-grounded, acupuncture for control of pain is being tried more often by western doctors.

IV

Game 7.12: Close your eyes and hold your right hand out in front of you, the index finger extended. Now, touch your right index finger with your left index finger. How many tries did it take? Put your right hand behind your back as far away from your body as you can and do the same thing. There is no need to close your eyes this time. Does it take more tries, the same number or fewer? Most people find that there is no significant difference.

Your ability to locate your index finger without seeing it illustrates proprioception, the sensing of one's body. In addition to the position-sensing neurons associated with muscles and tendons in the head, limbs and joints, proprioception includes chemical sensors, especially in the lungs and

gut. Data about chemical sensing is sometimes called intero-
ception.

Game 7.13: To illustrate chemical proprioception, hold your
breath for fifteen seconds. The pressure to breathe that you
feel is due in part to the build-up of carbon dioxide in the
blood.

Normal breathing allows the carbon dioxide carried away
from cells by the blood to be exchanged in the lungs for fresh
air including oxygen. If the exchange stops, chemical sensory
nerve endings in the lungs, blood vessels and the hind-brain
signal that normal breathing must be resumed. It is the
presence of carbon dioxide rather than the absence of
oxygen in the blood that first signals the need to breathe.
    Balance is also a form of proprioception, but it depends
on two elaborate, highly specialized sense organs, the vestibulary system in each ear. Balance actually consists of two
senses: gravity and acceleration.

Game 7.14: Ask a friend to whirl around as fast as possible.
He should keep his eyes open. Stop him when he is facing
you and watch his eyes. The pupils will drift in the direction
opposite to the direction of spin and then snap back again
into the middle. The drift may recur several times until your
friend has recovered his balance.

This phenomenon is a reflex action called nystagmus. It permits the eyes to remain fixed on an object even though the
head is moving, and it speeds up or slows down in direct
relation to the speed of movement.
    The mechanism responsible for the reflex consists of three
tiny semicircular canals in the bone just above the inner ear
(see Figure 7.4). They lie at roughly right angles to each
other. A chamber called the utricle connects the openings
of the canals to another chamber, the saccule, which in turn
opens into the cochlea, that portion of the inner ear which
contains the sound-sensing organ. All of the linked hollows
of the inner ear are filled with fluid. Towards the middle

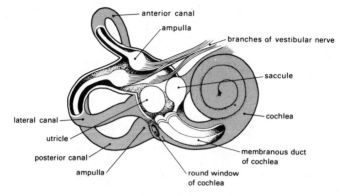

Fig. 7.4: The vestibulary system

of each semicircular canal the walls enlarge to form a ridge, or crista, which partially blocks the space. The crista surface is lined with neurons, their hairlike dendrites held in a gelatinous mass called the cupola which rests on the crista, nearly completing the closure of the canal. When you turn your head, the fluid moves in a direction opposite to the direction of turn. The fluid movement causes the cupola to swing like a flap, and the neurons in the crista signal this movement to the brain. The mechanism gives information about acceleration and deceleration and because of differences in the angles of the three canals, it also indicates angle of movement. If movement continues at the same rate and angle, however, the fluid stops moving and the cupola flops back to a neutral position – further evidence that the sensory apparatus favours whatever is new. Vision and proprioception then take over the job of conveying the movement data essential to balance. Sudden deceleration causes the cupola to flop in the opposite direction and may produce a sensation called reverse vertigo.

Gravity sense is the work of the utricle and saccule in each ear. They contain a gelatinous membrane in which calcium has been deposited. This otolith is attached to hairlike dendrites so that it moves in the chambers. When the head tilts, gravity pulls the otolith. A tilt to the left causes the otolith in the left ear to pull more than the one in the right. If you stand on your head, both otoliths record maximum pull.

Disturbances of the sense of balance cause feelings of vertigo and dizziness. The accompanying nausea occurs because there are connections within the brain to the vomiting centre in the hind-brain. These symptoms can be produced by different diseases, but one of the most common and least serious is motion sickness.

Game 7.15: You can produce all the feelings of seasickness by pouring or gently squirting cold water into your ear, but the water should not be too cold. If it feels cold on the hand, it is quite cold enough. Before you play this game, do remember that the symptoms of seasickness are most unpleasant.

This procedure demonstrates that motion sickness is not all in the mind. There is a physiological mechanism underlying it. Small children and animals can experience motion sickness. With sufficient provocation, indeed, everyone can be made to feel it.

Yet there can be no doubt that motion sickness is in part a conditioned response. The person who feels sick as soon as he steps on a boat is not responding to a disturbed mechanism of balance. A bout of sickness creates tension when the person next confronts a boat, plane or car. Children will often outgrow car sickness though they may continue to suffer air or seasickness.

As every victim knows, there is no cure. Drugs may help if they are taken at least thirty minutes before the motion begins. The most common drugs are antihistamines which cause drowsiness. After taking any anti-motion sickness pill, you should not drive for at least eight hours.

V

Almost two centuries ago the German physicist, George Simon Ohm, stated that the ear acts as an acoustic analyser; that is, it separates two or more different frequencies when they impinge on it. The same Ohm gave his name to the old unit of electrical resistance. The eye·uses the opposite approach with light: instead of separating, it synthesizes light frequencies making colour vision possible (see Chapter 8).

Game 7.16: You can test Ohm's acoustical law with two glasses and two spoons. Fill one glass with water so that it makes a high note when you strike it. Only part-fill the other so that it makes a low note. Now, hit the two glasses simultaneously with the two spoons. With a little practice you can resolve the single sound into its two components. Instead of glasses of water and spoons, you can use a piano or a guitar.

The ear can pick up frequencies from 20 to 20,000 cycles per second. Cycles per second, cps, are also called Herz (Hz) after the German physicist, H. R. Herz.

Game 7.17: You can obtain a very high frequency sound by turning on your TV and turning the sound down. You may be able to hear a high-pitched whine which equals about 16,000 Hz. If your hearing acuity has been reduced either by age or by damage to the auditory nerve, however, you may not hear the sound.

Obviously, the human ear is an astonishingly sensitive instrument if it has not been overstressed by excessive noise. The eardrum responds to air movements as small as one-tenth the diameter of an air molecule.

Ear structure has been traced back to the earliest fish in which the bony labyrinth, now the inner ear, first appeared. The cochlea developed in the early amphibians, and reptiles possess the three bones of the inner ear.

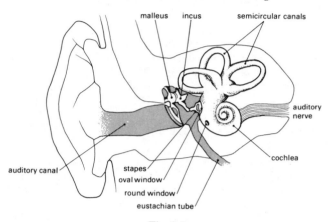

Fig. 7.5

The auditory canal of the outer ear concentrates the sound waves, approximately doubling their energy. In the middle ear the three bones, or ossicles, again double the force of vibration at the eardrum. The relative smallness of the oval window, the membrane at the entrance to the inner ear, compared to the ear drum further amplifies sound waves (see Figure 7.5).

The outer and middle ear contain air at normal pressure, maintained in the middle ear by the Eustachian tube which opens in the throat. In a jet plane or a fast lift, outer air pressure often falls or rises rapidly causing a temporary difference between air pressure outside and inside the eardrum. Your ears pop when you swallow or yawn to equalize air pressure in the middle ear. The inner ear, including the vestibulary system, is filled with a saltwater-like fluid which is not compressible.

The spiral cochlea is aesthetically the most beautiful of the sense organs. It is divided into three compartments running the entire length of the spiral. The two outer compartments are called the vestibulary and tympanic canals, respectively. Each is separated from the middle ear by two membranes, one at each end of the canals. Because of their shapes, these membranes are called the oval window and the round window. Vibrations set up in the fluid at the oval window end with concomitant fluctuations in the surface of the round window which relieve the fluid pressure after it has passed over the basilar membrane. The basilar membrane and Reissner's membrane (named after Ernst Reissner, German anatomist) surround the third cochlear compartment, the cochlear duct. The duct is not in contact with the middle ear, and it ends at the tip of the cochlear spiral, the helicotrema. The basilar membrane is about three centimetres long. Reissner's membrane becomes enlarged in the cochlear duct to form the tectorial membrane. This membrane contains tiny hairs which are extensions of specialized neurons forming the organ of Corti (after Alfonso Corti, Italian anatomist). This is the actual organ of sound sensing, analogous to the retina in the eye. It consists of about 23,500 cells which convert the mechanical energy in the inner-ear fluid to action potentials. The entire length of the organ of Corti rests on the basilar membrane, and it is the movement of this membrane which moves the hair cells. Fluid pressure causes the basilar membrane to undulate in relation to the frequency of the sound waves. Higher frequencies produce a wave peak near the oval window. Lower frequencies cause undulations to travel the length of the basilar membrane with wave peaks much further away from the oval window. This differential is reflected in the activity of the hair cells so that cells nearer the oval window signal higher frequencies and those at the other end, lower frequencies. Each neuron in the organ of Corti seems to be tuned to a very limited frequency range. The electrochemical process by which mechanical energy from the basilar membrane produces a neuronal action potential is not understood.

Game 7.18: The skin on the inside of your forearm has about the same resiliency and elasticity as your basilar membrane. You can demonstrate how different frequencies are fairly specific in their effect on the basilar membrane by using your forearm as a sounding board. High frequency peaks early and has a relatively localized effect. An electric razor with a vibrating head produces a high frequency vibration. Place the razor lightly against the forearm skin just above your wrist. The vibration should be felt only near the razor head. Now, rest your forearm lightly against a source of low frequency vibration, for example, a washing machine in operation. The vibration will seem to travel the length of your arm.

Axons from the cells of the organ of Corti form the auditory nerve. In the hind-brain, signals from each ear are split so that half go to the opposite hemisphere and half remain on the same side. The limited frequency tuning applies to successive neurons in the pathway, and the arrangement of frequencies from high to low found on the basilar membrane is roughly maintained both in the superior colliculi, where cells respond to light as well as to sound signals, and in the auditory cortex. In the medial geniculate moreover, where the last synapse takes place before the auditory cortex, there are cells which signal in response to signals from the 'correct' frequency cells but are inhibited by the 'incorrect' frequencies. They behave like the on-off regions observed in the touch sensors and in vision. The primary auditory cortex is in the deep sulcus dividing the temporal from the parietal lobe, roughly inside and just above each ear.

8 Sensation II: Seeing

I

More is known about the machinery of vision than about the other senses. Perhaps one reason is the easy isolation of the eyeball. Though you cannot remove your eyeball, you can demonstrate that it has a remarkable range. Despite its location in a bony socket at the front of your head, you can see behind your back.

Game 8.1: Look straight ahead. Hold your right arm straight out to your side and reach backward keeping your arm straight. Keep your head absolutely fixed to the front but turn your eyes in the direction of your arm. Wriggle the fingers on your outstretched hand (movement is most easily seen) and move the arm slowly forward – keeping it straight – until you can just glimpse your fingers. Bend your arm at the elbow only, moving your hand towards your forehead but keep your arm and hand in the same plane in which you first saw your fingers. Your fingers should hit your temple just behind your eye.

When they are open but not busy, your eyes move constantly. They make tiny involuntary movements, called saccades, which you do not usually notice.

Game 8.2: To observe saccades you must have a very dark room where you can fix your eyes unmovingly on a dim light source, for example, a lighted cigarette end fixed about six feet away from your face. After a short time, the cigarette end will appear to jump.
   The eye tends to drift off centre. When some critical point is exceeded, an order to involuntary muscles brings the eyes

back to the fixation point. The brain centre responsible for this control is in the upper quadrant of the frontal lobe just in front of the sensory-motor homunculus, a location at some distance from the visual cortex to which it must nevertheless be connected.

Game 8.3: It is possible to observe similar eye movements if you watch the eyes of a reader whose head remains still. The text he is reading must also be still. Ask a friend to sit in a good light, reading a book or paper placed on a slanted platform so that it is possible for you to see his eyes. He is not to move his head at all, but to read normally. You will see that his eyes do not move continuously across the page. They seem to jump. This movement too is regulated by the eye-movement region in the frontal lobe. Though it is normally involuntary, it can be brought under voluntary control. One of the exercises used to improve reading speed, for example, is to try to take in more words in the printed line without eye movement.

The eyeball itself is completely independent of its socket and is connected to the body only by the optic nerve and blood vessels (see Figure 8.1).

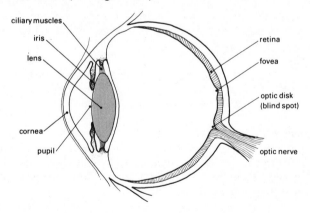

Fig. 8.1

Game 8.4: You can observe your own retina, or more precisely, the blood vessels which feed it. In a dimly-lit room shine a small, bright flashlight through your closed eyelid. The shadows of the retinal blood vessels will be picked out by the light.

These blood vessels run through the retina as well as across its inner surface. The rest of the eyeball serves to collect and focus light on to the retina, the light-sensing organ. It is unique among sense organs because it develops in the fetus as an outgrowth from the brain itself. The retina covers roughly three-fifths of the back surface of the eyeball. It consists of three layers of neurons. The innermost are called ganglion cells, and it is their axons which form the optic nerve. Next to them, towards the outer margin of the eyeball, is a layer consisting of three types of cell called bipolar, amacrine and horizontal. Outside this layer, oriented away from the light source, are the light-sensitive cells, the rods and cones. Light enters through the cornea and passes through the vitreous humour, a clear jelly, which fills the eyeball. The thickness and shape of the lens is regulated by the muscles forming the iris. The light then passes through the retinal blood vessels and the three neuronal layers to the choroid, the inner membranous shell of the eyeball. The choroid surface is pigmented so that it stops light, like the silvering on the back of a mirror, and serves as a reflector, throwing the light forward again on to the rods and cones.

There are some 100 million rods and only about 6 million cones in the human retina. Both are distributed across the entire surface, but a major concentration of cone cells is to be found in the fovea at the retinal end of the optical axis. The fovea is a pit filled with cone cells surrounded by a small circle of yellow-pigmented cells called the macula lutea.

Game 8.5: You can observe your own macula lutea with a piece of white paper, a bright light and a piece of dark blue or purple cellophane. Shine the light on the white paper and look at it with one eye closed. Quickly bring the cellophane between your open eye and the paper. In the middle of the paper you should see a faint circular shadow for a second or two. The shadow is your macula lutea. Its yellow pigment absorbs blue light from the cellophane leaving a grey shadow. If a quick look through the cellophane fails to produce the shadow, move the cellophane towards and away from your eye a few times, keeping it between your eye and the brightly-lit paper. Or you can look at the blue sky on a cloudless summer day. You may briefly see the same circular shadow. Indeed, the shadow was first noticed by the British physicist, James Clerk Maxwell, in just this way and is still called Maxwell's spot.

In the fovea there are no cell layers above the cones. Because the cones operate most efficiently with bright light, the fovea is the point of highest resolution or acuity.

Game 8.6: Figure 8.2 is designed to illustrate the high resolving power of the fovea. With your right hand hold the diagram about six inches in front of your right eye. Note that six inches is very close to your eye indeed. Cover your left eye with your left hand. Look at the + at 0 degrees. The letter S above it will be clear. The A at 5 degrees should be legible, but the other letters will probably be fuzzy or unreadable. You are looking at the + very closely so that it falls almost alone on your fovea.

Near the fovea there is another pit in the retina. It has no receptor cells at all because it is the place at which the optic nerve leaves the eyeball. It is a blind spot.

Game 8.7: You can also observe your blind spot by using Figure 8.3. Close one eye. Hold the book about 12 to 15 inches in front of you and look at the square. Move the book towards you and away until you find a position at which you can no longer see the +. The image of the + is now falling directly on your blind spot. Note that the line seems to be continuous. Nor do you see a 'hole' in

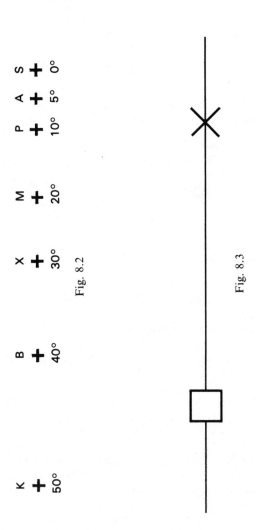

K +
50°

B +
40°

X +
30°

M +
20°

P +
10°

A +
5°

S +
0°

Fig. 8.2

Fig. 8.3

nature. This is an interesting perceptual phenomenon in which you are automatically supplying the sensory data missing because of the blind spot.

The rods dominate all parts of the retina outside the macula lutea. They are sensitive to motion in dim light. At night one can often see more clearly by looking out of the corner of the eye rather than straight ahead because of the concentration of rods at the periphery of the retina.

Game 8.8: On a blank piece of typing paper place a black dot in the middle of one of the shorter edges and a black line along the other shorter edge. Hold the paper sideways about 12 inches in front of you and fixate the dot. The line at the other end of the sheet should be just visible when you begin, but it will slowly fade. If you shake the paper without otherwise moving it while continuing to fixate the dot, the line should reappear. The rods at the periphery will have picked up the motion.

Rods and cones contain chemicals called visual pigments. The pigments are opsins, chemically-related to vitamin A, the carrot vitamin, out of which the opsins are synthesized by the rods and cones. In the rods the visual pigment is called rhodopsin. In the cones it is a slightly different chemical, iodopsin. There are three different varieties of iodopsin, moreover, and each cone contains only one.

The three varieties of iodopsin are the chemical basis of colour vision. One is particularly responsive to light in the blue wavelength, one to green light and one to red. With these three colour responses the average human eye can detect 200 hues. If one variety of iodopsin is deficient, we suffer colour blindness for that colour. However, colour vision depends to some extent on learning and is more complicated than the description of three chemicals implies.

In both rods and cones the opsin molecules are arranged in discs, several thousand of which lie stacked one on top of the other in the specialized dendritic ends of the cells. When the visual pigment receives light, it is changed chemically in such a way that a flow of ions begins in the neuron. Thus, light energy is converted to electrochemical energy in the form of an action potential. When bright or continuous light causes all or a large number of the opsin molecules to change chemically, the cone or rod is temporarily 'blinded'. This is visual adaptation (see Chapter 7).

Game 8.9: Visual adaptation can be observed in the afterimage. With a bright light shining on the page, stare at Figure 8.4 for a minute. Now, shift your gaze to a well-lit whitish wall or to a blank sheet of white paper. You should see, towards the middle of the field of vision, a light spot about the size of the spot in the figure. It is an after image.

Fig. 8.4

The bipolar, amacrine and horizontal cells forming the middle layer of the retina collect the signals from rods and cones. Some of these cells excite the inner layer of ganglion cells and others are inhibitory. They begin the definition of retinal fields. As against some 100 million rods and cones, there are only about half a million ganglion cells, and their axons form the optic nerve. Thus, the grouping of signals into retinal fields starts visual data processing before light sensation reaches the brain.

Ganglion cell behaviour has been explored by the standard neurophysiological procedures. A microelectrode is inserted under anesthesia into the retina of an experimental animal until the action potential of one cell can be observed.

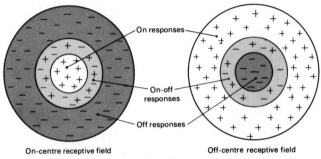

On-centre receptive field   Off-centre receptive field

Fig. 8.5

That cell is then exposed to a stimulus: the signals from a group of rod and cone cells. Two kinds of ganglion cells have been detected. One is an on-centre cell, the other an off-centre cell. These curious names refer to the nature of the receptive field – the group of rods and cones – served by the ganglion cell. Both types of cell are represented in Figure 8.5. Light falling on rods and cones at the centre of the field excites the ganglion cells to signal. Light falling on cells immediately surrounding the central receptors may have no effect, but light falling on cells at the periphery of the retinal field is inhibitory. It turns the ganglion cell off. The off-centre ganglion cell works in the opposite direction.

Game 8.10: That these on-off fields are probably repeated in the visual cortex where we sense their effects can be illustrated if you stare at the grids in Figure 8.6. Grid (a) is called a Chladni figure. Stare at one intersection and note that dark dots appear at all intersections in the figure except the fixation point. The on-centre receptive fields illustrated in (b) could explain this illusion.

Now stare at each of the two grids containing intersections of varying sizes. In the black grid (c) the dark spots are more easily seen in the thin intersections, though they can also be observed in the thick intersections if that grid

Fig. 8.6: The influence of black and white areas on on-centre receptor fields (based on Frisby, *Seeing: Illusion, Brain and Mind*, 1979): (a) top; (b) centre; (c) bottom left; (d) bottom right

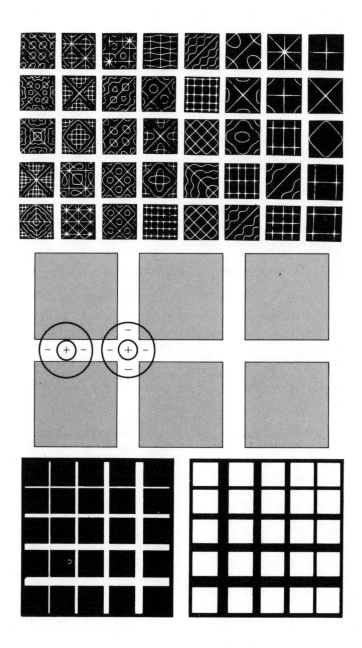

is held further away from the eyes. The black intersections (d), with their illusory white dots, probably reflect the operations of off-centre retinal fields.

The retinal ganglion cells may also signal at different speeds so that some signals reach the brain more quickly than others. We might reasonably guess that peripheral rods detecting movement synapse with fast ganglion cells, but this is speculation.

The optic nerve enters the skull and runs beneath the forebrain to meet at the optic chiasma (crossing) just outside the brain. At the chiasma, the fibres forming the two nerves divide. Those from ganglion cells with fields in the outer half of each eye – the half furthest from the nose – go to the brain hemisphere on the same side as the eye where they began. Those from the inner half of each eye go to the opposite hemisphere. Because the lens reverses the image that falls on the retina right to left and upside down, the right visual field is projected on to the inner or nose half of the retina of the right eye and the outer half of the left eye. Conversely, the left visual field is projected on to the inner half of the left retina and the outer half of the right. In this way the whole visual field goes to each side of the brain. The optic nerves end in centres in each hemisphere called the lateral geniculate nuclei. The retinal fields are retained in the geniculate nuclei, as are the on-centre, off-centre signals. Lateral geniculate cells also seem to respond specifically to signals originated by one colour and to be inhibited by other colours in a manner analogous to the on-centre, off-centre cells.

One group of neurons run from each lateral geniculate nucleus to the superior colliculus on the same side where the visual map is juxtaposed to auditory and touch maps. The largest group of neurons leaving the lateral geniculate, however, run to the primary visual cortexes at the backs of the occipital lobes – right at the back of the head. In the visual cortex the number of cells is greatly multiplied again to something like the original number of rods and cones. These arrangements and the functions that arise because of them have been the subject of some of the most remarkable research conducted by biologists in the second half of the century. As with all scientific research, it began a long time ago, but the major landmarks in understanding the visual cortex were built by two groups of American scientists.

In 1959 J. Y. Lettvin, H. R. Maturna, W. S. McCulloch and W. H. Pitts, at the Massachusetts Institute of Technology, published a paper with the graphic title, 'What the Frog's Eye Tells the Frog's Brain'. Using microelectrodes in the frog's visual cortex (actually, the colliculi in frogs), they were able to locate four types of neurons both in the retina and in the brain. One type detects and responds to edges; that is, contrasts between light and dark. Type two sees 'net convexity', corners or rounded dots – like flies. The third type also detects edges, but only if they are moving. Finally, there are 'net dimming receptors'. They respond only to a 'sudden reduction of illumination by a dark object'. It takes very little imagination to see how these four types of receptor meet a frog's needs. More important, the research showed that specific cells play specific roles, at least in the visual system of frogs.

In another brilliant series of experiments in the 1960s, using apes, D. H. Hubel and T. N. Wiesel of Harvard explored the cells of the mammalian visual cortex. Not surprisingly they found more than four types of receivers, which they grouped under three broad headings:

1. Simple cortical cells include (a) Dark-line detectors in specific orientations; one cell will respond to⸺ but not to ╱ or | . (b) Bright-line detectors, also in specific orientations, and (c) Edge detectors in specific orientations.
2. Complex cells which detect motion. Some cells signal in response to motion in either direction, and some to motion in only one direction. Some respond only if the received signal is in a specific orientation, analogous to 1(a) and some have no preferred orientation.

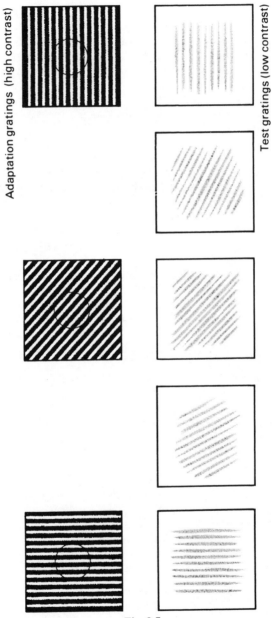

Fig. 8.7

3. Hypercomplex cells include length detectors; that is, cells that respond to___but not to_____. There are also width detectors and angle detectors.

Hubel and Wiesel found evidence that all of these cell types are arranged in columns running through the cortex. Each column appears to contain all the different cell types, and the columns are juxtaposed forming maps of the visual fields.

Now by playing a few games we can explore psychological effects which demonstrate the existence of the kinds of cells Hubel and Wiesel described.

Game 8.11: In Figure 8.7 the gratings on the left are high contrast and each contains a circle. The grating lines are all of the same width and the contrast in each is the same, but their orientations differ. These are the orientation adaptation gratings. The gratings on the right are low contrast, and their orientations change across a compass quadrant from 90 to 0 degrees. These are the test gratings. Note that they can be seen only faintly.

Select one of the adaptation gratings and stare at it for at least a minute. During the adaptation period move your eye around within the circle. This will avoid an after image (see Game 8.9). After the adaptation period look at the appropriate test grating: 0 degrees for the vertical adaptation grating, 90 degrees for the horizontal adaptation grating. You should find that you can no longer see the test grating or the grating with the angle closest to it, but you should have no difficulty seeing the other test gratings as before adaptation.

Let us say you have used the top, vertical adaptation grating. What has happened is this: the simple cells for this orientation have become tired. In electrochemical terms this means a reduction in the frequency of action potentials in the neuron. The reason for this is not clearly understood, but as a result when you look at the vertical test grating, it has disappeared. Cells with orientations near the vertical

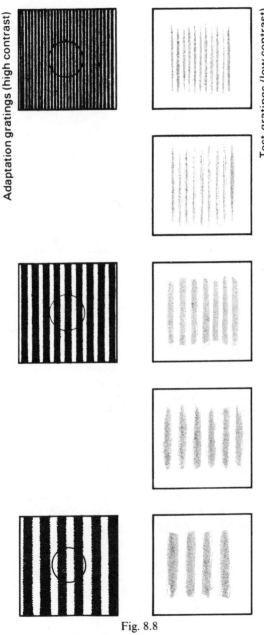

Fig. 8.8

are also affected but less so. Those responsive to horizontal signals and to angles near horizontal have not been adapted, and these test gratings are still visible.

There are not many behavioural tests which demonstrate so effectively the correctness of neurophysiological data. For good reason gratings have been called psychological micro-electrodes. Your performance on grating tests may improve with practice, suggesting that learning plays some role in the activities of the visual cortical cells. This intriguing possibility is discussed at the end of this chapter. For the present we can look at more gratings.

Game 8.12: The gratings in Figure 8.8 demonstrate the existence of width receptors.

Game 8.13: The gratings in Figure 8.9 can be used to demonstrate size adaptation, but they also reveal an illusion called the tilt after effect. Note that the middle test gratings have the same contrast as the adaptation gratings. The adaptation in this game will produce an after-effect illusion

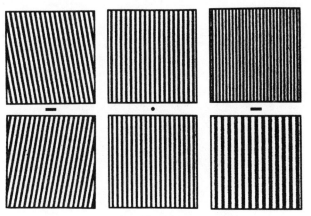

Fig. 8.9

in the centre test gratings rather than the adaptation blindness in the two preceding games. The dot between the test gratings provides a fixation point when you return your eyes to them after adaptation. The short thick lines between the adaptation gratings are for fixation during adaptation. To

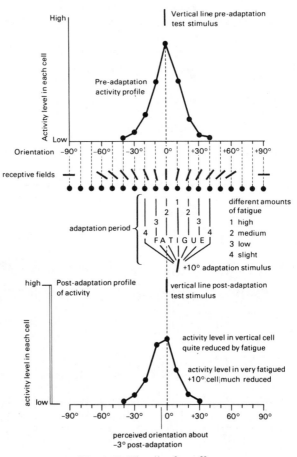

Fig. 8.10: The tilt after-effect

avoid an after image, move your eyes the short distance back and forth along their length.

Try the tilt after effect first. Stare at the line between the left-hand gratings for at least a minute. Now fix upon the spot between the vertical test gratings. They should appear to tilt, but in the opposite directions to the tilts of the respective adaptation gratings. Figure 8.10 helps us to see why.

For simplicity the figure assumes that you have been looking at just one line instead of a grating. Note the receptive fields of the simple cells in the middle of the figure. Above them the curve shows their activity when you first look at the vertical test gratings. Now assume one adaptation grating with a tilt of $+10$ degrees, as shown. During adaptation the $+10$ degree-oriented cells tire most, the vertical- and 20-degree-oriented cells next, and so on, as shown in the numbers above the word *fatigue*. When you look back at the test grating, the bottom curve shows what is happening to your line orientation cells: the $+10$ degree cell activity is much reduced and the vertical cell activity is also down. The -10 degrees cell activity, on the other hand, is hardly reduced at all. Therefore, it signals the vertical line relatively more strongly than the vertical-oriented cell itself (by comparison with the pre-adaptation activity profile), producing an illusion of a tilt to the left.

Now return to the width-adaptation gratings. After adaptation, you should find that the top test grating appears to consist of thicker lines than the bottom one. The explanation is similar to the explanation of the tilt after effect.

Game 8.14: Turn to Figure 8.11. Cut the page along the dotted lines. Cut a hole in the centre of the spiral to accomodate the spindle of your record turntable. Place the spiral on your turntable and turn it on at 33⅓ rpm. Stare at the centre of the rotating disc for about a minute. Turn off the record player. You should see the spiral rotating in the opposite direction. Readapt to the rotating spiral; that is, turn on your record player again and stare at the centre of the spiral for another minute. Shift your eyes quickly to some well-lit flat surface such as a desk top. You should see the illusory reversed spiral moving in the desk top!

We shall return to this marvellous perceptual illusion in Chapter 9. It demonstrates that we are capable of seeing a logical impossibility: the spiral in the perfectly visible desk top. Apparently, the visual system can detect two attributes quite independently of each other, and it is 'happy to live with a paradox'.

The neural explanation of this remarkable after-effect recalls the existence of movement detectors. Theoretically, they must be operating in pairs in what is called an opponent-process system. The most likely model of such a system was proposed by an Austrian physiologist, Sigmund Exner, in 1894 – three-quarters of a century before Hubel and Wiesel described movement detectors. Exner suggested that two neurons record movement right and movement left respectively, and that they are paired. Presented with a stationary object, both continue to emit background noise only – that is, occasional random action potentials – and the observer therefore perceives only the stationary stimulus. Then the stimulus – the spiral – is observed for a minute moving to the right. The right movement neuron signal becomes dominant because it is excited while its left movement twin continues to emit only occasional random signals. At first, the right movement neuron signals very rapidly, but as it becomes fatigued, it signals more slowly and finally stops altogether. Now the moving stimulus stops. The right movement neuron is too tired to emit even random signals at first, but the left movement neuron, quite unimpaired, does signal at random. It becomes the dominant twin until the right movement twin recovers. During this period lasting about 20 seconds, the stationary stimulus seems to move to the left.

An analogous effect can be obtained if you stare at a waterfall for a minute or two. If you then shift your gaze to the riverbank, it will at first appear to move upwards.

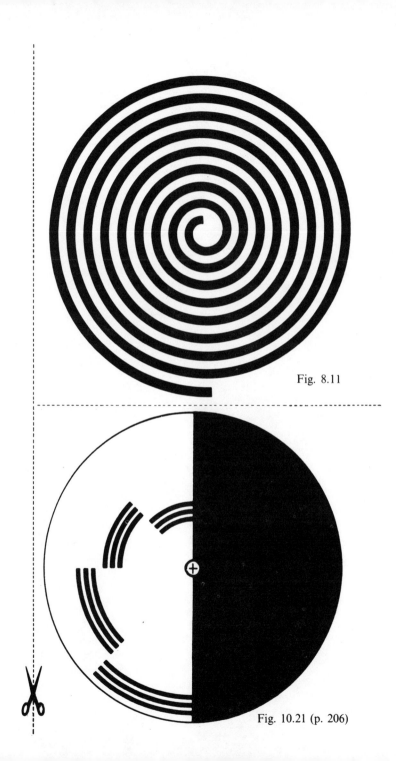

Fig. 8.11

Fig. 10.21 (p. 206)

You will find several more of these perceptual games in Chapter 9. Let us continue with illusions that reveal the nervous mechanisms of vision.

Game 8.15: You will need a large white piece of paper set in a blotter pad with wide black or brown edges. Place it on a table or desk top. You will also need a good light source such as a desk lamp with a 100 watt bulb shaded so that the light shines on the desk surface. Place the lamp at one end of the desk and turn it on. What you see is pretty obvious: a dark surface with a white square bounded by a blotter pad, all brightly, if unequally, lit by the lamp at one end.

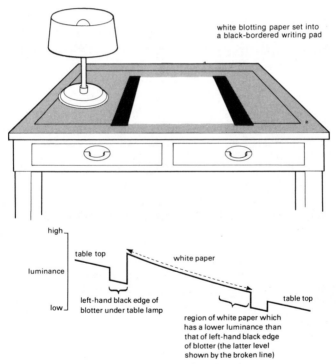

Fig. 8.12: Analysis of luminance

Yet if you consider the luminance of the surface, defined as the amount of light falling on it (illumination) and the proportion bounced off it (reflectance), Figure 8.12 shows what a tricky problem your visual system has analysed.

The left-hand blotter edge near the light is seen as black or brown despite the fact that its luminance is greater than the luminance of the other end of the white paper. We compute lightness correctly because the reflectance from the table top is the same across the entire surface. We can see a brightly or dimly lit white, as against a brightly or dimly lit black, for the same reason that we do not see the blind spot in the retina: we fill in the correct data. In part this ability may be learned, and in that case it would have to be considered to be a perceptual trick rather than a neurophysiological phenomenon per se. Yet you will remember that there are edge detectors in the visual system, and the American psychologist, Dr Edwin Land, suggested how they can explain the luminance illusion. Land was also the inventor of the first polaroid camera.

Game 8.16: Study Figure 8.13. At first glance A and B look alike, a light grey area abutting a dark grey area. Look at their luminance profiles in C and D, however, and you will see that they are quite different. A does consist of one dark grey block next to a light grey block, but B consists of two blocks of exactly the same grey excepting that the right-hand block contains an edge at the middle. You can be certain about this if you lay a pencil along the boundary within B.

This illusion is called the Craik-Cornsweet-O'Brien illusion after the three British psychologists who discovered it. It probably occurs because C and D are observed by edge-detecting neurons responding to straight edges between dark and light. A has a real edge, but the luminance in B is shown by D to be higher at the boundary than elsewhere in the block. E and F show how edge detectors respond, and G and H, how our visual equipment fills in the rest.

In both hemispheres many different specialized detectors arranged in columns form a map of the retinal fields. Depth

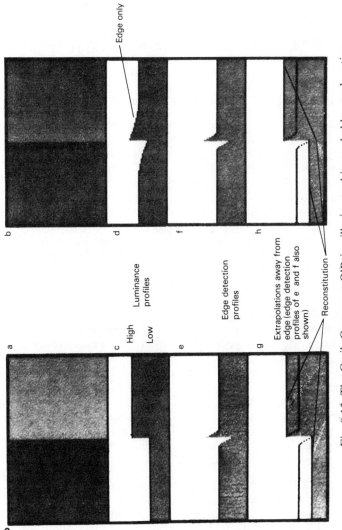

Fig. 8.13: The Craik-Cornsweet-O'Brian illusion and its probable explanation

perception results from the stereoscopic vision provided by the slightly overlapping field from cells responding to light from each eye.

Game 8.17: Hold a pencil directly in front of your nose, horizontally with the end nearest you slanted slightly downwards. Open and close each eye alternately. The pencil will appear to swing through an arc. With both eyes open you can see the pencil straight ahead of your nose.

Game 8.18: Hold two pencils, one vertically in each hand, at arm's length in front of your face. Try to see the pencils and not your hands. Now move them alternately towards your face and away. Note the depth. This test, incidentally, is similar to one used by the United States Army Air Force during World War II to measure depth perception. The two pencils were sticks in short tracks at the end of a square, lighted tunnel. The subject looked at the sticks through a hole at one end of the tunnel opposite the short tracks. With two strings, one attached to each stick, he had to pull the sticks until they appeared to him to be even. If he saw them at the same depth when they were in fact more than 5 centimetres apart, the subject was unable to train as a pilot. It was considered that his faulty depth perception would endanger his ability to land a plane successfully. There is some evidence, however, that subjects could improve their scores by repeated use of the apparatus. Perhaps we learn to use other clues such as luminance for depth perception.

In Game 8.18 the two pencils keep their respective sizes despite changes in the size of the images they cast on the retina. This phenomenon is called size constancy. It is perceptual, like the filling in of the blind spot, and not a function of neuronal machinery.

Game 8.19: Hold one hand at arm's length directly in front of your face. When you move it in and out, there is of course no change in its apparent size. Now keeping your arm and hand outstretched, hold the other index finger about 10 inches from your face. Fixate the finger, but keep your hand in view. If you now move your hand in and out, it will appear to grow and shrink. The loss of size constancy seems to result from the diversion created by your index finger.

This game and illusions such as the Craik-Cornsweet-O'Brien luminance illusion raise a question: Is the specialized function of an individual neuron an inherited phenomenon, or is it learned in some degree? The English neurophysiologist, Colin Blakemore, working with several other scientists in various experiments, has been in the vanguard of those whose research suggests that a high degree of learning may be necessary for neuronal specialization to become operative. For example, in one experiment with G. F. Cooper, Blakemore reared kittens in darkness except for a short period each day when some of the kittens were placed in a drum the inside of which was painted with vertical black and white stripes. A large paper ruff was fitted round the neck of the animal so that it could not see its own body, and the drum was then lighted. After several weeks of this experience, the cats were exposed to gratings with various orientations. As revealed by the signals picked up by micro-electrodes, the 'vertically-reared' cats lacked 'horizontally-specialized neurons'. Kittens which had been placed in drums with horizontal bars lacked vertically-specialized neurons. Some form of learning seems to be essential to the correct development of visual neurons, at least in cats.

Infants born with a squint in one eye are known to lose their capability for binocular depth perception unless corrective measures are taken very early. The defect in depth perception could be caused by the squint which inhibits proper development of certain neurons. In any event, birth defects in vision are now given immediate attention in order to counteract their influence if possible before the post-natal period of neuronal development ends.

There is another intriguing phenomenon suggesting that learning plays a role in the development of human visual machinery as it appears to do in cats. Studies have shown that Caucasians have a greater sensitivity to vertical and horizontal gratings than to oblique gratings. Most Caucasians see vertical and horizontal gratings with lower contrasts whereas the contrasts in oblique gratings must be stronger before these subjects can see them.

Game 8.20: Using the test gratings in Games 8.10 to 8.12, see how this applies to you. You will have to estimate your sensitivity to the different orientations, but do not assume that your skin colour will determine your reactions. Read on.

There could be several reasons for such a visual preference. The vertically- and horizontally-specialized neurons may be more sensitive than those tuned to obliques, or there may be more of the vertically- and horizontally- specialized cells, but there is no evidence to support either theory. It is also possible that we see verticals and horizontals more easily because our environment consists of vertical buildings with horizontal rows of windows and floors, in which case there would be no apparent reason for the phenomenon to be limited to Caucasians. Yet this possibility gains support from the fact that Asians living in Asia show no preference for vertical and horizontal gratings against oblique ones. In part of course the difference between Asians and Caucasians could reflect a genetic distinction which would produce a physiological difference. With the evidence now available, there is no way to decide between a physiological and an environmental explanation except to repeat again that neuronal machinery appears to be unaffected by geography; that is, no one has ever demonstrated racial differences in the wiring. In any case visual preference is a problem of perception which is a product of experience. First, therefore, we must take a quick, unemotional look at the emotions.

9 Emotion

I

Game 9.1: P A P E R
When you saw the word above, what image was the first to come to your mind? Did you think of a book page, a paper napkin, art paper, toilet paper?

Whichever image you saw when you read the word, it came to you because of the feelings you were having when you began to read this chapter. Perhaps your feelings had to do with the reason why you picked up the book when you did. Perhaps they resulted from a sense of well-being in a warm room, or perhaps a quarrel, or a business worry. Think for a moment whether the first image you saw might have been different had your mood been different.

You saw the word 'paper', a sensory event reflecting physical phenomena. You interpreted the marks on the page as a word with a meaning because you had learned at school to do this. But the image you saw was influenced by your emotional state. In short, your perception was influenced not only by sensation and experience but also by emotion.

Emotion and motivation are, of course, closely related, even if the words do not mean exactly the same things. Fear is both an emotion and a powerful motivation. Behaviourists prefer to call motivation a drive, partly because drive lacks the emotive quality of the word 'motivation'. Hunger is a drive. Certainly it is a motivation, but it is seldom described as an emotion. It can arouse strong emotions, though, like fury, despair and hatred. Perhaps it will be easier to forget about the distinction between emotion and motivation and to look instead at a possible difference in the origins of emotions.

On the one hand there are strong 'primitive' emotions, such as fear, anger and sexual desire, which humans share with other animals and which may be part of the inherited machinery. On the other hand there are the learned emotions, feelings which include love or hatred of a person or object, joy stemming from musical sounds or visual sensations. There is evidence that different parts of the brain are responsible for the two different kinds of emotion. As I pointed out in Chapter 2, stimulation of centres in the hypothalamus can produce feelings of pleasure, fear, anger or sexual desire as well as hunger and thirst. Learned emotions seem to be stored in part of the right frontal lobe. Thus the older emotions are controlled by the older part of the brain and the 'newer' emotions by the cortex.

There is another distinction that may be important because it, too, is based on your physiology. The next time you watch a horror movie on TV, note your physical reactions. I know this sort of self-analysis tends to spoil the film, but perhaps you can obtain a different kind of pleasure by acting in the interests of science! Your heart beats faster. You may sweat, especially in the palms of your hands and on the soles of your feet. Your mouth will go dry. You will feel a general sense of muscular tension. If you are watching with someone, look at their eyes – or use a mirror to look at your own. The pupils will be dilated. You will not be able to observe the constriction of blood vessels in your skin and the reduction of activity in your gut, but these two events also usually accompany fear or horror. All of these physical changes are evidence of the operation of one part of your involuntary nervous system, the sympathetic system. The body is being readied to fight or to run. A hypothalamic releasing factor may be assumed to have caused the pituitary to secrete ACTH and the adrenal glands are pumping adrenaline into the blood. In other words, the hypothalamus is backing up the involuntary nervous system with a chemical command which helps to mobilize the energy reserves needed by muscles in action.

At the opposite extreme are the reactions that accompany

emotions of pleasure and sadness or distress. You can check these changes too when you are watching a sad film. Your heart rate slows, your muscles relax and your limbs tend to flex. You will cry, or at least feel like it. Though again you cannot observe them, your peripheral blood vessels will have dilated and there may be increased gut activity. These are symptoms of calming rather than excitation. They indicate the operation of the other part of the autonomic nervous system, the parasympathetic. The symptoms of sadness could also be protective in that they counteract the grief born, for example, of bereavement.

The physical changes produced by strong emotions are themselves subject to cultural conditioning. For example, an Anglo-Saxon male watching a sad film is unlikely to allow his parasympathetic to activate his lacrymal glands. An Anglo-Saxon female, on the other hand, or a Mediterranean – male or female – is much more likely to cry. What we fear and what pleases or angers us, what tastes edible and what is sexually desirable – all such feelings are powerfully influenced by learning.

Game 9.2: This game depends on the pupillary reflex described in Chapter 3. You will need a large and varied selection of pictures culled from magazines, your own photographs or any other source. The pictures used in Games 3.3 and 5.8 will serve as a basis for this collection, which should include nudes as well as geometrical designs and abstractions. Number the pictures on the back so that you can see the numbers, and keep a checklist in front of you with a one- or two-word description of each picture. You will also need a friend to act as your subject. The object is to observe the effect of picture content on the size of your friends' pupils.

Let the subject look through the pictures at his own speed but without long pauses or repetition. Those which interest or excite him will produce noticeable enlargements of the pupils. You will find that the time he devotes to a picture may not be a good check; for example, he may pass more quickly over a nude because of embarrassment at his own feelings. The pupils alone afford an objective measure. If you mark on your checklist those items that cause your friends' pupils to enlarge, you should end up with a profile of his interests.

Tests of this kind have revealed that men's pupils enlarge more when they look at pictures of women with large pupils than when the pupils of the women are small. Apparently, we recognize that large pupils mean interest, and we respond accordingly. It has also been found that the pupillary response increases in hungry subjects.

Hunger can also influence memory.

Game 9.3: Ask two friends to help you with this game. Each is to memorize the following list of word pairs. You will time them to discover how long it takes from the time they begin until they have the list word-perfect.

fruit-apple	room-sofa
cheese-cracker	bed-window
pancake-steak	egg-stair
pie-ham	stew-ceiling
carpet-rug	house-butter
lamp-light	screen-potato

One friend is to memorize the list just before a main meal. The other should memorize it just after a large meal.

You should find that the before-dinner subject is faster than the after-dinner subject. The former will recall the words most easily. Incidentally, if you can, check their memories a day later. There should be no significant difference in their recall, a memory phenomenon for which there seems to be no clear explanation.

Tests on people of normal weight show that after they are given a glucose drink directly into their stomachs through a tube so that they cannot taste it, a sugar solution becomes unpleasant to the taste. You have probably experienced something like this when an excess of sweets makes the next one quite unpalatable, or when you eat too much of a fatty food you like. Such temporary changes in taste seem to demonstrate the operation of a satiety centre, a role played by yet another group of neurons in the hypothalamus. If the satiety centre is damaged or removed, experimental animals will continue to eat as long as food is available. It is interesting, therefore, that the sugar test does not work with many obese subjects. To them, the sugar solution may continue to taste pleasant even after their stomachs have been loaded with glucose. In these obese patients, there may be a malfunction of the satiety centre.

We have very little more hard evidence about how the emotions work or how drives are channelled in the brain and nervous system. Their power is perhaps all too obvious. Their effects can be seen again and again in the way we perceive. A simple test that provides you with an emotional profile may be useful.

Game 9.4: By answering the following sixteen questions, you can obtain a personal profile of your emotions. Score yourself between 1 and 5 depending on where you fit between the extremes. You may also like to score a friend and then compare your evaluation to his self-judgement: but beware, this kind of game can lead to quarrels.

1   You have a date to go out with someone you like. At the last minute, the person phones to apologize and explain that something has come up. Do you
  lose your temper? (1)
  accept the apology without complaint? (5)
2   Do you
  fall in love too easily? (1)
  Have you
  never been in love? (5)
3   It took me___try(ies) to pass my driving test.
  One (5)
  Five (1)

4 You are hammering in a nail in an awkward place and hit your finger. Do you

   lose your temper? (1)

   carry on as smoothly as your injured finger permits? (5)

5 A lady has just collapsed in the shop where you work. There is no one else in the shop. She looks very ill. Do you

   panic and yell for help? (1)

   dial 999 and ask for an ambulance? (5)

6 You are inching your car slowly along in a double line of heavy traffic leaving plenty of space between you and the next car. A driver behind you sounds his horn to make you close up the gap. Do you

   stop and angrily get out to remonstrate? (1)

   move forward to close up the gap? (5)

7 You are facing away from the room door. You are sitting comfortably reading with the radio on excluding other sounds. Suddenly, you look up to see a friend standing in front of you. Do you

   jump and cry out? (1)

   welcome your friend and turn off the radio? (5)

8 You are chatting to another parent in the street. You turn to discover your five-year-old standing on the curb some distance from you. Do you

   yell at the child and run towards him? (1)

   call the child quietly and walk towards him with your friend? (5)

9 You are awakened by a noise in the house. Do you

   cower in your bed too frightened to move? (1)

   wait to identify the noise before quietly taking action? (5)

10 The white sauce curdles and within seconds the soup boils over. Your dinner guests are already at the table. Do you

   panic? (1)

   turn off the soup and pour out the sauce preparatory to making it again? (5)

11 The thought of Hitler, the Ayatollah Khomeini, Begin,
Qaddifi or Mrs Thatcher makes you
   furious. (1)
   consider their motives and how to change them. (5)

12 You discover your eight-year-old child exposing him-
or herself to a child of the same age. Do you
   slap your child and send the friend home? (1)
   ignore them? (5)

13 You are on the top floor of a hotel when the fire alarm
sounds. Do you
   panic? (1)
   pull on a few clothes and look for the nearest fire
   escape? (5)

14 You happen to be looking at a book your neighbour
on the bus is reading when (he) (she) turns a page to
reveal a photograph of a sexual act. Do you
   look away and move your seat when you can? (1)
   continue to look? (5)

15 Your mate suggests that you try a sexual act that is
new to you. Do you
   shudder and turn away? (1)
   try it? (5)

16 You are sailing as crew with an experienced friend. A
sudden wind squall pushes the boat on to its beam.
Do you
   feel panic and wish to be anywhere else? (1)
   brace yourself and wait for the squall to pass? (5)

Add up your scores in four groups:
Anger questions: 1, 4, 6, 11
Sexuality questions: 2, 12, 14, 15
Composure questions: 3, 5, 8, 10
Fear questions: 7, 9, 13, 16

Add up your scores

The minimum score for each of the four emotions is four,
and the maximum, twenty. A score near the minimum of

sixteen indicates a high degree of emotionality. A score near the maximum of eighty indicates very little emotionality.

When you think about your score on this game, bear in mind that your emotions influence not only what you choose to sense and do, but also that they reflect an integrated system of physical states involving hormones as well as nervous mechanisms. Now, think what might happen if you were to repress an emotion, or perhaps to live as though you felt something which you did not feel. Have you been taught to 'swallow your anger', to 'avoid excessive display', to mask your emotions? Very few of us have not. Repression might well countermand the physical orders issued by your hypothalamus impeding the natural anger, for example, which produces a releasing factor causing the pituitary to secrete ACTH, and so on. Clearly, a neurosis or, at the least, stomach ulcers might be the result. Yet most of us get away with such repression every day and suffer only minor physical symptoms such as an occasional headache. It is a tribute to the flexibility of our physiological balances that usually no more goes wrong. But our physical ability to accept the need for occasional repression is also recognition of a vitally-important fact: we are social animals with an unusually well-developed capacity to foresee the results of our behaviour. It is for this reason that culture – any culture – offers us great rewards in exchange for self-control; rewards that make occasional repression literally easier than that will-o-the-wisp, doing one's own thing. Because the cultural rewards for self-control are so high, our physiological systems are reset by experience like a thermostat in a cold house. Emotion affects the sensations we perceive within the context of experience.

10   Perception

I

Saturday night and Sunday morning may both be warm and moonlit, but they never feel the same. Nor does darkness if you are alone compared to being with a lover.

Emotion affects perception. At two weeks an infant recognizes and prefers a human face to any other face. Soon afterwards it is the mother's face the infant prefers.

Similarly learning, memory and sensation affect perception.

Perception is, in a sense, unconscious thought. The British psychologist, Richard Gregory, calls it a 'kind of problem solving'. A thing is perceived as distinct from being sensed when it is recognized and fitted into a system of familiar associations. If you see a flower which you do not recognize, you nevertheless catalogue it as a flower, perhaps as 'flower: unrecognized; to be looked up'. A. R. Luria pointed out that even one's perception of oneself grows out of emotion, experience and sensation. From studies with illiterate peasants in Azerbaijan during the 1930s, he wrote, 'we found critical self-awareness to be the final product of socially determined psychological development, rather than its primary starting point, as Descartes' ideas would have led us to believe.' Four hundred years ago René Descartes set down his axiom: 'I think; therefore, I am.' Nor is it only scientists from Communist countries who think that the reverse of Descartes' argument is probably closer to the truth.

Game 10.1: For this game you need a friend and either a metronome or a clock with a loud tick which can be muffled at will, say with a tea cosy. Your friend will be the subject because you will know what is supposed to happen.

Tell your friend that he is to listen to two sets of clicks separated by an interval of two or three seconds. He is to tell you whether the two sets have the same or a different number of clicks.

The first set should consist of exactly ten clicks at intervals of about a second. The second set should consist of either nine, ten or eleven clicks with the same intervals. You should find that your friend is almost never wrong. He may not be able to tell you how many clicks he heard, at least not when you start the game, but he can almost always tell you whether the number of clicks were the same or different. In other words, your friend perceived the pattern rather than the content. However the pattern originates, whether genetically or culturally, it gives meaning to the sights and sounds amongst which we live.

Game 10.2: Figure 10.1 shows an ink blot of the sort found in the famous Rorschach test. Study it and write down what you see. Put your analysis away where you can find it. This game is to be continued (on page 226), but I will not tell you how just yet.

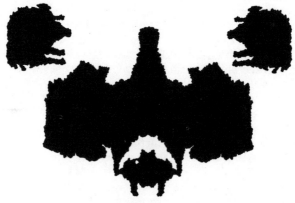

Fig. 10.1

Herman Rorschach was a Swiss psychiatrist who held that the patterns a person finds in random images tell something about his personality. He developed ten ink blots in all, two with a second colour (red), three with pastel colours and five black and white. Rorschach's ink blots are too diffuse and allow too great a diversity of interpretation to be a consistent guide to personality, and yet there is evidence from other sources that he was right in supposing that there is a loose connection between interpretation and personality.

Game 10.3: There are three patterns in Figure 10.2. Decide what each one looks like and write down your answers. Now turn the page.

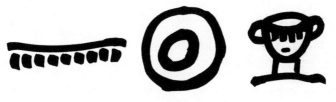

Fig. 10.2

Statistically, the answers by women differ from those by men. Unless you are prepared to argue the proposition that women inherit visual apparatus that works differently from men's, a proposition impossible to prove, the reasons for the differences in Games 10.3 must be cultural. Such cultural differences in perception can be made even more explicit.

Game 10.4: Figure 10.3 is called the 'devil's tuning fork'. Study it for about half a minute. Close the book and immediately draw what you saw. Compare your finished drawing to the figure.

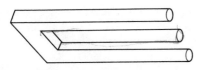

Fig. 10.3

> **Game 10.3, continued:** Responses to the three patterns differ statistically according to the sex of the observer. Most men see something that differs from what most women see. Most men see the left-hand figure as a brush or centipede. Most women see it as a comb or as teeth. Men see the middle figure as a target; women as a dinner plate. (Statistically, the same number of men and women identify the middle figure as a ring or as a tire.) The right-hand pattern is seen by men as a head; by women as a cup.

Most readers will have great difficulty with the drawing, even though they have read the name given to the figure. You interpret it as a three-dimensional representation and try to draw it accordingly, whereas like all illustrations in ink on paper, it is in fact two-dimensional. The trouble with your three-dimensional representation is that it contradicts the ambiguous depth cues in the figure.

Your compulsion to see the figure in three dimensions is a cultural phenomenon. Africans who have not received a formal education have no difficulty in drawing the figure. They see it merely as a series of lines and not as something solid. That one acquires the capacity to see three dimensions in a flat figure is also suggested by drawings produced by children and by many schizophrenics. I am not implying that uneducated Africans are 'like' either children or schizophrenics. For very different reasons, our cultural training has not affected the perceptions of these three groups of people.

This argument should be carried into art, however, only with the greatest care. It probably does not apply, for example, to the two-dimensional art of ancient Egypt or to the Saxon stone carvers or the twelfth-century Sienese painters. These artists may not have been conscious of perspective as a technical skill, but they certainly understood the principle of three-dimensionality. If they were unable to reproduce it in their work as perspective, they did so by means of an agreed iconography which their viewers understood to mean three dimensions.

II

Having established the role of culture in perception, we must circumscribe any inclination to make the environment play an absolute role. The tendency to perceive a rhythm or pattern rather than the details of an experience is universal. Out of the myriad stars scattered across the heavens, men have made constellations – patterns which have no reality in astronomy but exist for the observer, particularly for the traveller for whom the stars are a guide. There is reason to believe that pattern-making underlies all perception in a manner which implies some physical component.

Game 10.5: Look at the perfectly symmetrical grid in Figure 10.4. After you have stared at it for a few seconds, you will probably begin to see patterns of squares. They are not there, of course, but this involuntary grouping is hard to stop.

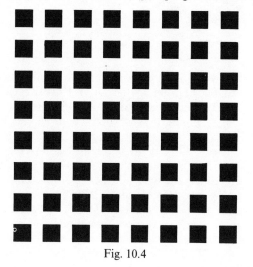

Fig. 10.4

Game 10.6: Look at the collection of dots in Figure 10.5. How long does it take you to discover the object hidden in the dots?

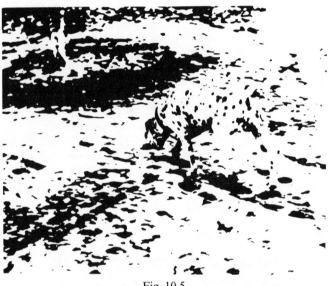

Fig. 10.5

A British psychologist named Kenneth Craik (the man whose surname appears in the Craik-Cornsweet-O'Brien illusion) observed that the brain makes models in the same way as we play games. It asks 'what would happen if', and then searches for an answer. Engineers draw plans for a bridge before they try to build it. Neuropyschologists advance theories summing up the facts and thus suggest experiments to test the theoretical design. In order to catch a train you have to have an idea about how you are going to get from your house to the station and how long it will take. You make a mental space-time model of the journey.

Models allow thought as we know it. Incidentally, Craik died in 1943, aged thirty-one. He was knocked off his bicycle in Cambridge by someone carelessly opening a car door, and run over. The irony of such a terrible accident merely adds point to Craik's insight.

Game 10.7: Figure 10.6 shows a computer program for the second player in a game of noughts and crosses. It can be beaten. Try it.

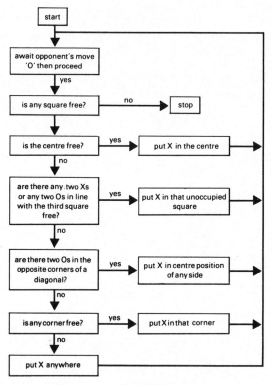

Fig. 10.6

The program is a model. Note that it is written down in ordinary language. In the machine the program would probably appear as a series of on-off switches. In either case it can be translated into numbers; for example, 0 for on and 1 for off. The model language must be learned, but perhaps model-making is one of the attributes of brain structure.

During the 1920s, a group of European psychologists opposed to the mechanical simplicity of behaviourism proposed that the brain inherits certain formal relationships. Gestalt (German: form) psychology correctly observed the tendency to build models and tried to analyse the component parts of that tendency. Gestalt psychologists looked for the basic forms model building might use. Three spatial relationships without cultural influences seem to them to be inherent in perception.

Proximity is illustrated in Figure 10.7. Most observers group the pairs in three vertical columns.

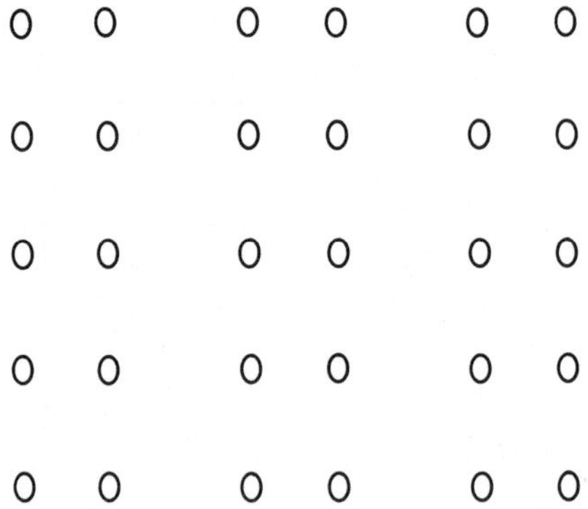

O   O   O   O   O   O

O   O   O   O   O   O

O   O   O   O   O   O

O   O   O   O   O   O

O   O   O   O   O   O

Fig. 10.7

Similarity causes us to see vertical rather than horizontal lines of dots in Figure 10.8.

Common fate describes the condition in which things move together in the same figure at the same time as in Figure 10.9.

In addition four other spatial qualities are considered by the Gestalt psychologists to be universal formal elements of the human brain. Set and habit are hard to distinguish

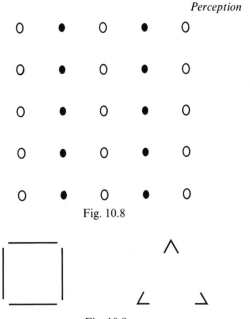

Fig. 10.8

Fig. 10.9

from each other, and both appear to be founded in experience. Direction and closure can be distinguished from common fate only with great care. Using these organizational principles, the mind cleans up a visual stimulus by making it consistent and 'whole', according to the Gestaltists.

Game 10.8: You will need paper and pencil for this game. Look quickly at Figure 10.10. Do not linger over it, but turn the page quickly and try to reproduce what you saw.

Compare your drawings to those printed in Figure 10.10.

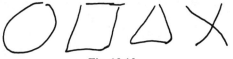

Fig. 10.10

Be careful. Did you notice that the round figure is an ellipse tilted to the right and not a circle? Did you notice and reproduce the break in it? Did you see that the square has no right angles, and that the 'triangle' has two round corners and an open end? Does your drawn X consist of two curved lines like the printed figure? If you missed some or all of these points you have demonstrated the Gestalt theory that the organizational principles in your mind caused you to clean up the figures. You obeyed the Law of Pragnanz.

The notion of in-built form is no more absurd than the notion of linguistic deep structures (see Chapter 6). Indeed, it could be much sillier to reject such inherited traits. Science is about discovering the simplest explanation for any event, a rule often identified as Ockham's razor. As usual, the difficulty is the absence of concrete evidence that these formal attributes do somehow exist in the neuronal machinery.

Yet the slate is no longer totally blank. New evidence shows that specific neurons do respond to specific associations. A British neuropsychologist, E. T. Rolls, reported in 1980 the discovery of three such specialized regions in different parts of the brains of primates, each of which is connected to the visual cortex. In the monkey hypothalamus, he found neurons which signal in response to the sight of food, but not to other objects. Thus, an apple produced an action potential but a rubber ball did not. Rolls does not know whether this is a learned or an instinctual response, but it is significant that a perception – of an *edible* object has an identifiable physical foundation.

The second region Rolls found is close to the hippocampus and the thalamus. Here, neurons fired in response to a familiar visual stimulus but not to a novel sight. In the experiment an animal was taught to recognize an object, let us say a large red rubber ball. The ball would then be seen to produce a neuronal response whereas a small black ball would not. Nor would these neurons signal in response to general visual stimuli, such as the room in which the experiment was conducted. They seem to incorporate a specific recognition, but that is not quite the same as saying they contain a memory of a large red rubber ball.

Finally, in a part of the sensory-motor cortex connected to but not in the visual cortex, Rolls found neurons that clearly discriminate between two familiar visual stimuli. They would not signal at the sight of food or drink or balls, but they did signal when the animal was shown a face. It could be either a human face or a monkey face of any size or colour, upside down or at 90 degrees, though some neurons failed to respond if the face was in profile! There

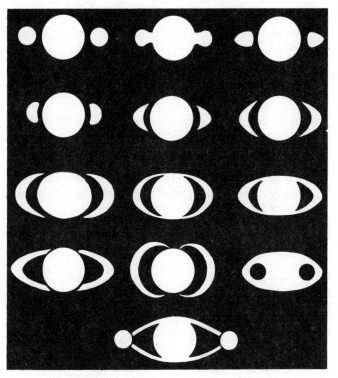

Fig. 10.11: Huygens's drawings of Saturn

seemed to be no emotional association. The neurons responded whether the animal was angry or contented, but facial features such as the eyes did make a difference. There was no response at all from these cells when the eyes were covered. Other neurons in this group responded also to hair, mouth, teeth or to several different facial features, as well as to the whole face. Some signalled only in response to the whole face. These astonishing facial neurons show how specific perception could be. They do not include the Gestalt forms – so far – but it is clear that neurons which respond to faces or to familiar objects have significant survival value.

In order to identify an object such as a face correctly, there must be some sort of an internal model to compare it with; what Richard Gregory has called an 'object hypothesis'. In his book, *The Intelligent Eye*, Gregory reproduced the original drawings of the planet, Saturn, made by the Dutch astronomer, Christiaan Huygens (see Figure 10.11).

The drawings show the astronomer's misinterpretation of Saturn's rings which, Gregory suggests, is the result of an erroneous object hypothesis. Sometime later Huygens realized that the simplest explanation of what he saw through his telescope was a 'thin, flat ring, nowhere attached to the body of the planet.' The television pictures sent back to earth by the Explorer satellite in 1980 show that even this intelligent guess is an approximation.

Game 10.9: Here is a problem in perception which requires an object hypothesis to obtain a solution. What does Figure 10.12 show?

The answer requires that you distinguish figure from ground; that is, what is object and what is background, or

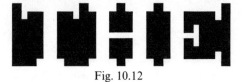

Fig. 10.12

in the language of communications, what is signal and what is noise.

Game 10.10: Read this line:
    socks some brought who wet

Now read this line:
    who brought some wet socks

The difference between the two lines can be described as a reduction in noise. The second is obviously slightly easier to read.

Game 10.11: Figure 10.13 is a visual figure-ground problem. The Greek vase illusion was first published in 1915 by a Danish psychologist, Edgar Rubin. The reversal – the vases and the pair of faces – requires a shift in the definition of figure and ground, respectively.

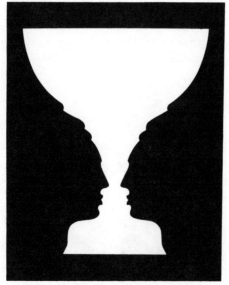

Fig. 10.13

Game 10.12: Ambiguous figures illustrate a similar image reversibility. Figure 10.14 is by Gerald Fisher. To the left, a man's face. To the right, a weeping girl. In the middle ... ?

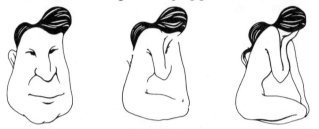

Fig. 10.14

Game 10.13: By far the most difficult, for me at least, is the ambiguous mother-in-law created by the American psychologist, E. G. Boring (see Figure 10.15).

It is impossible to see both of the images in Games 10.11 to 10.13 at the same time. Yet they are undeniably both there. Your attention is somehow drawn to one or the other,

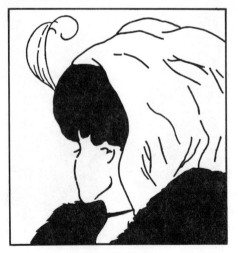

Fig. 10.15

and you may then have to exert an act of will to force a shift. At the least you will have to blink or glance away from the figure to obtain the reverse image.

III

One of the most interesting illusions created by the noise arising from ground is called the Fraser spiral.

Game 10.14: In Figure 10.16, follow any part of the curve carefully with your finger or a pencil. What do you find?

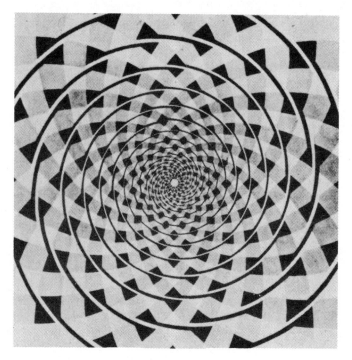

Fig. 10.16

Be sure to keep your finger exactly on the curve you began to follow and accept that seeing is not necessarily believing.

The Fraser spiral does not move, nor does the spiral in Game 8.13 after the record player has been turned off. Yet both are seen to move under suitable conditions.

Game 10.15: Take a heavy piece of white or near-white paper and fold it along the long axis, thus

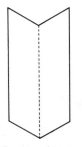

Set it up on a flat surface at about chest height, thus

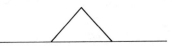

Stant directly in front of the fold. Select a spot in the middle of the fold (do *not* mark the spot), and look at it steadily with one eye shut. At first it should resemble Figure 10.17.

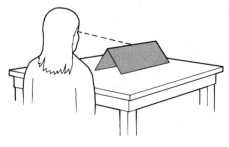

Fig. 10.17

Continue to stare at the folded paper. It should suddenly 'stand up', as in Figure 10.18. When the folded paper stands up, move your head slowly back and forth but continue to stare at it with one eye. It should appear to twist and turn.

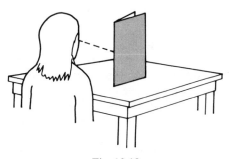

Fig. 10.18

This curious double illusion demonstrates a phenomenon called motion parallax. When you first see the folded paper, it is lying down and you see it lying down. All the depth information and the light and shadow are consistent. When it stands up, the cues are contradictory, and when you move your head, the fact that the near point of the fold crosses the retina before the far point causes the image to appear sinuous. This is another example of the 'impossible' perception ascribed to the sensory apparatus in Chapter 8.

When we perceive an object actually in motion, the signaling by visual cortical neurons is quite different. Actual motion produces signals in those neurons most attuned to movement in the direction of the motion, but if you take a still photograph of a moving object using a 125 millimetre shutter speed, the image will be smeared. We do not perceive smearing when we look at a rapidly-moving object, such as a diver or a football in flight. The object looks whole and steady, in part because we have a theory or model of space which takes account of objects moving through it. The perception of movement assumes that the ground is still.

Game 10.16: The next time you take a train ride, try to observe again the familar motion illusion which occurs when you are stationary and a train beside you moves off. The reverse illusion can occur when your train moves off leaving another one standing. In both cases balance, touch and hearing cues quickly put you straight.

Game 10.17: Draw a line about ½ inch long on a small piece of white paper. Hold the paper directly in front of your nose at a distance of eight to ten inches. Close each eye alternately. The line should appear to be displaced because of the separation between the two eyes. If you wink each eye alternately fairly rapidly, the line will seem to move. This is called stroboscopic, or phi, movement. The illusion is the basis of movies and television, and the next game illustrates the principle. It was first performed in the eighteenth century with an ember tied to a string.

Game 10.18: Tie a small flashlight to the end of a stout string. Turn the flashlight on in a dark room or outside on a dark night and whirl it around. You should see a continuous line of light rather than a series of images.

From the speed reached by the light when it is perceived as a line, it has been estimated that the electrical activity of rod and cone cells lasts from 150 to 250 msecs, roughly one-fifth to one-quarter of a second. Motion pictures are projected at the rate of twenty-four to thirty frames per second. To prevent a flicker the light beam is interrupted once or twice during the flashing of each frame. Television images are actually painted on the screen as a series of horizontal lines. The most common image now consists of 525 lines. Each line is made up of about 500 dots. The complete image is presented thirty times per second. If you can manage to see any of the systems conveying printed information on a television screen, you can watch each frame being constructed line by line and letter by letter. This is a slowed-down analogy of the way the usual TV picture is built up.

Game 10.19: The English neuropsychologist, Horace Barlow, has suggested this demonstration of another illusion of movement. You will need a bright light source shaded so that only a vertical bar of light about six to eight inches wide is thrown on a screen. You will also need a bar or a solid foot rule about an inch across. Place the bar across the light source so that its shadow reaches from edge to edge of the light and move the bar up and down. At the correct speed, which will vary with the width of the bar and of the light, the bar will appear to bend in the middle. The ends will turn upwards as the bar comes down and downwards as it goes up. The probable explanation is that the outer edges of the dark bar are dimmer than the centre. The images from the ends of the bar may take more time to stimulate retinal rod cells and could reach the cortex after the blacker image from the centre of the bar.

Motion takes place within space and is part of the theory of space. We have already examined three-dimensionality as part of that theory, but now we can look again at perspective within which motion occurs.

Game 10.20: Lay a piece of paper beside the nearest of the three cylinders in Figure 10.19. Mark the top and bottom points. Now lay the measure against the other two cylinders. How do you explain the result?

Game 10.21: In Figure 10.20 there are no straight lines extending into the distance. Nevertheless, you will almost certainly see a platform full of barrels.

Why should two-dimensional ellipses becoming smaller look like a real scene? The figures in this and the preceding game employ the same principle as the devil's tuning fork in Game 10.4. We see depth because of experience, and we accept that motion occurs within three-dimensional space for the same reason. Note that it was not always so. The Ptolemaic universe, for example, posited the heavens as one curved plane through holes in which the light of stars

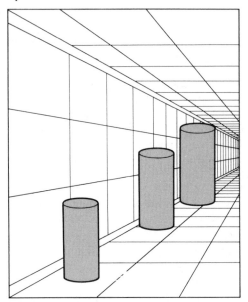

Fig. 10.19: Equal or unequal cylinders?

shone. This two-dimensional image of the movement of the heavenly bodies appears in many renaissance paintings before Copernicus, Brahe and Galileo created the three-dimensional object hypothesis with which we still live.

Another set of illusions underlies our perception of colour. Our sensory apparatus conveys sensations of three discrete wavelengths, as we have noted, but it can be tricked.

Game 10.22: Figure 10.21 on p. 171 shows Benham's top. It was invented as a toy in 1894. Cut it out and mount the pattern on a piece of card. Punch a hole through the centre point marked + and insert a nail or pencil. Holding the top upright on a flat surface, spin it. Colours should soon appear. If you spin it clockwise, red should appear towards the centre with a band of yellow around it encircled by green with blue or violet on the outside. If you spin it counter-clockwise,

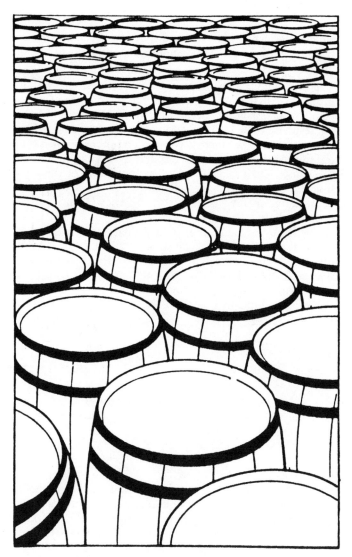

Fig. 10.20: Two-dimensional or three-dimensional?

the order of the colours should be reversed with blue or violet at the centre and red on the outside. If you are colour-blind, the colour that you cannot see normally will still be missing.

This marvellous illusion is not fully understood, but its probable explanation begins with the three types of visual pigments in cone cells. Because of the wave nature of light, the response of neurons to colour depends on differing time constants; that is, each wavelength requires a tiny time difference for its reception. The curved grids on the Benham top cause light flashes to occur at the speeds of the three time constants. The cone cells and their specially-attuned connections in the visual cortex are tricked into sensing coloured light.

The illusion of colour is actually part of everyday life. From three visual wavelengths we build up the familiar diversity of hues. Depending on whether the colour is additive, as in beams of coloured light, or subtractive, as in ink or paint, we perceive colour mixtures in accordance with the two diagrams in Figure 10.22.

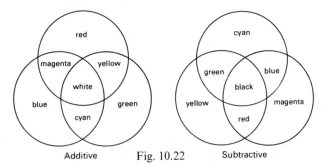

Additive   Fig. 10.22   Subtractive

Game 10.23: You will need three flashlights and three pieces of cellophane coloured red, blue and green respectively. You may also need a friend to hold one of the flashlights. Play with the coloured lights. You are mixing colours in the way that stage and film lighting technicians do.

Subtractive colour perception can be achieved by painting

with watercolours. Or you can see how the trick is achieved if you will look at a painting by Seurat. Instead of mixing the paints on his palette, Seurat applied tiny dots of colour in patterns so that at a distance the spectator's eyes do the mixing.

IV

Perception is affected by the physical quality of adaptation which we discussed in connection with the visual system (Chapter 8). Of course, adaptation affects all the senses.

Game 10.24: You will need three bowls of water. The left-hand bowl should contain hot water (about 90 to 100 degrees F); the right-hand bowl, cold water (about 60 degrees F) and the middle bowl tepid water. Put your left hand in the hot water and your right hand in the cold. When they have both adapted and feel about the same, put both hands in the middle bowl. The left should feel warm and the right cool.

This trick was first described by the English philosopher, John Locke, in 1690. To Locke it demonstrated that temperature is all in the mind. He was only partly wrong, as we know. There are neuronal receptors sensitive to temperature (Chapter 7), and there is a temperature-sensitive region in the hypothalamus. Yet Locke was right about the perception of temperature. If the water is hotter than about 105 degrees and colder than about 60 degrees, however, the perception of pain will probably precede adaptation.

Game 10.25: You will need a radio or record player with a volume control separate from the on-off switch. Just before you go to bed, set the machine at a comfortable volume level and turn it off. When you awaken, turn it on without moving the volume control. It should now sound noticeably louder than it did the night before. During the night your auditory nerves have recovered from the adaptation that took place during the day.

Game 10.26: Press your arm against a wall for about a minute. When you move away, your arm will feel light and may even tend to rise a few inches. The touch receptors and proprioceptors have adapted to the pressure, and your arm muscles temporarily overcompensate.

Game 10.27: Make a fresh solution of water and sugar. Hold it in your mouth for a minute. Spit it out or swallow it and immediately take a mouthful of fresh water. It should taste slightly salty because the sweet receptors have adapted.

There is a similar perceptual condition called habituation. Whereas adaptation is a psychological perception of neuronal activity, however, habituation has no physiological foundation. It is a concomitant of attention and is, therefore, influenced by learning. For example, you are unaware of a clock ticking in the room until it stops. You may sense the touch of your clothes for the first few seconds after you put them on, but as habituation intervenes perception of the sensations stops. By the time you have read this far, though, the chances are that you are again aware of the feel of your clothes.

Game 10.28: You will need a stopwatch or a clock with a sweep second hand or one that records the seconds digitally. You will also need the help of a friend. When you awaken in the morning, count to sixty at what seem to you to be intervals of one second. Your friend is to clock you and to record the actual time covered by your counting. You should not see the actual times until the game ends. Repeat the counting and timing throughout the day whenever it is convenient. The last time should be just before you go to bed.

You will probably find that your counting in relation to clock time becomes faster as the day passes. This shortening of perceived time may be caused by the rise of about one degree in your body temperature which normally takes place during the day. As body temperature rises, metabolism (all the activities of cells) may increase slightly because higher temperatures tend to hasten chemical reactions. The various so-called body clocks based upon cellular activities would then speed up. One's perception of clock time would be over-estimated, and time would tend to pass more slowly.

Although with practice it is often possible to awaken at a predetermined hour (see Chapter 3), you are almost totally unaware of the passage of time during sleep. Psychoactive drugs also affect the perception of time. Hallucinogens like LSD and marijuana and even tranquillizers cause it to slow down relative to clock time, perhaps by causing perceptions to become extended. Amphetamines can cause time to speed up because amphetamine is a stimulant. You can test the effects of drugs on perception with nothing stronger than tea or coffee.

Game 10.29: Figure 10.23 is called a Necker cube. When you look at it steadily, the points marked A and B may be seen to reverse their orientation. A will be nearer at first and B further away. Then B will seem nearer and A will be further away. Of course, the two points are equidistant. Your experience of perspective causes you to see depth in the figure. The reversal occurs because the perceived

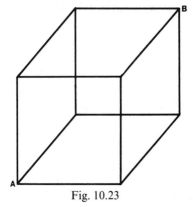

Fig. 10.23

perspective contradicts the two-dimensionality of the figure. This illusion is similar to the one noted in Game 10.15.

Now, drink a cup of strong tea or coffee. Wait a quarter of an hour and repeat the experiment with the Necker cube. You should see more reversals than you did before. The stimulant (caffeine in coffee, caffeine and theobromine in tea) apparently speeds up the process of perception as well as the contradiction that goes with it.

We have no neurons specialized for sensing time directly. After all, time is not a natural phenomenon. Duration occurs in nature, but time is man-made. The significance of time varies greatly from pre-technical to technical cultures and even within a single culture. If you are a stickler for promptness and your friend is always late, you have an example of what I mean.

Duration is often cyclic in nature: the moon, the seasons, day and night. Not surprisingly, animal physiology is conditioned by the natural cycles. Because many cells have their own rhythms, it is fashionable to talk about biological clocks. Some of them are indeed related to external natural rhythms. The estral period is closely related to the moon cycle. The cycle of sleep and waking is related to day and night, though experiments with men in caves have shown that this clock can be reset with relatively little experience. On the other hand, the renewal of skin cells is not cyclic, nor even regularly periodic. Cell functions wax and wane at different rates, and evidence for a central time-keeping mechanism in the brain analogous, for example, to the temperature-regulating centre in the hypothalamus is controversial. Perhaps it is not surprising that the hypothalamus is in fact the prime candidate for the role of central time-keeper.

Perception of time is not necessarily related to any physiological clock. In general the more that is going on, the more rapidly time seems to pass. The less that is going on, the slower time passes. These generalizations fit experience with sleep and with drugs, and they also apply to reaction time.

Game 10.30: You will need a deck of cards and a stopwatch or a clock with a sweep second hand or with digitally-displayed seconds. Sort out the sixteen cards, ace, 2, 3, 4 in all suits. Then, sort out sixteen cards consisting of two of each of the 5s, 6s, 7s, 8s, 9s, 10s, Jacks and Queens. Shuffle each pack of sixteen separately. Take the sixteen cards, ace to 4, and sort them into piles by number. Time the operation accurately. Now, do the same with the sixteen cards, 5s to Queens. You should find that the second set of sixteen takes longer to sort, probably because you are having to cope with more different stimuli. You will probably not have noticed any time difference precisely because you were dealing with more stimuli.

Though there is no time receptor as such in the nervous system, some people are much better than others at guessing what time it is. They are usually those who do not customarily wear a wrist watch. Probably, they learn to use other cues such as changes in light. They may also have learned to perceive time intervals whereas those of us who wear a watch depend on that machine.

VI

When all is said and done, perception remains as mysterious as consciousness. Somehow action potentials in the brain, evoked by sensations, stimulate memory and emotion to produce psychological responses. Some physiological data exist, as we have seen, but they are tantalizing rather than conclusive. One of the most mysterious aspects of perception is how it seems to work, often quickly and accurately, with very little sensory data.

Game 10.31: Read this:

Thxs, wx cax drxp oxt exerx thxrd xetxer xnd xou xtixl mxnaxe pxetxy wxll. Thng ar a litl toghr i we ls leve ut he pac. Anevnwrsifecnnctheors.

If you get lost, there is a translation on the following page.

> **Game 10.31, continued:** Thus, we can drop out every third letter and you still manage pretty well. Things are a little tougher if we also leave out the space. And even worse if we connect the words.

But you will probably have read the whole message with only minor delays. All that you needed – in addition to the ability to read English – was the rule: drop every third letter.

An American computer specialist, O. Selfridge, has proposed a model based on what we know about the power of perception and about brain function that makes sense. He called his model Pandemonium. Figure 10.24 was re-drawn from one by Leanne Hinton for an American psychology textbook, *Human Information Processing* by Peter H. Lindsay and Donald A. Norman.

Pandemonium consists of a series of demons each of whom does a different job. The Image Demons have the simplest jobs. Like the retinal rods and cones, they record the image. Next, Feature Demons note the straight lines, the angles and the curves, like the visual cortical cells with their specialized functions. Now, we find a large and mysterious population of Cognitive Demons. Each one is responsible for one learned phenomenon; thus, the twenty-six letters of the alphabet are represented by twenty-six Cognitive Demons. In theory, if the model is correct, a memory for each letter is encoded in a neuron or neuron net somewhere in the brain. Probably the 'face' and 'familiarity' neurons fall into this class (see p. 196). The Cognitive Demons note the features of the stimulus and shout when one is recognized. In the illustration F has two horizontal lines and P has a discontinuous curve, but only R recognizes all the features. R, therefore, shouts the loudest of all. Finally, there is a Decision Demon, one only, who listens to the pandemonium until he or she discovers who is making the most noise. The Decision Demon is you or me.

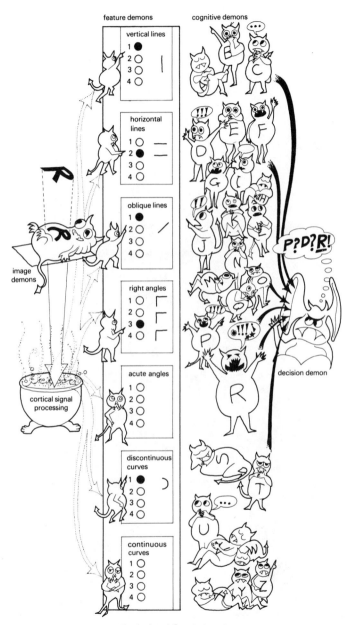

Fig. 10.24: Pandemonium

Afterword:
The Unhealthy Brain

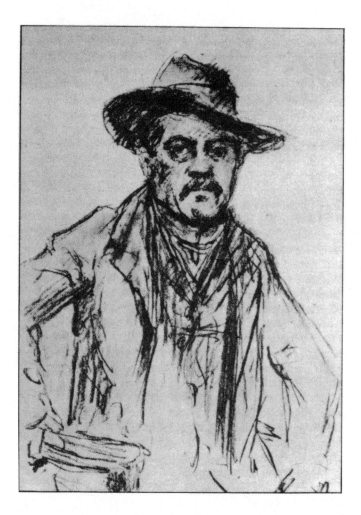

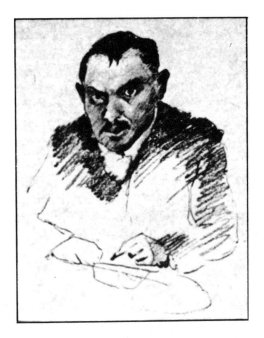

Lovis Corinth, the German artist who drew these two self-portraits was born in 1858. In December 1911 he suffered a severe stroke. A stroke is also called a cardiovascular accident. Blood supply to a part of the brain is impaired and the nerve cells die. Corinth's stroke affected his right hemisphere. He was much weakened on his left side, and he was left severely depressed.

When he began to work again, several months after the stroke, Corinth's style had changed dramatically. The first self-portrait is from the immediate pre-stroke period. The second was drawn soon after the stroke. Most art critics at the time assumed that the change reflected Corinth's illness and subsequent depression. They saw in the second self-portrait and many other pictures like it the artist's increased awareness of life's fragility and death's inevitability. Perhaps so, but the irregularity of the post-seizure contours, the misplaced details and the blurring of texture all suggest right hemisphere damage (see Chapter 2). These distortions are even more noticeable in Corinth's two portraits of his wife, Charlotte. Note that in the post-seizure portrait, the left side of Charlotte's face and body are

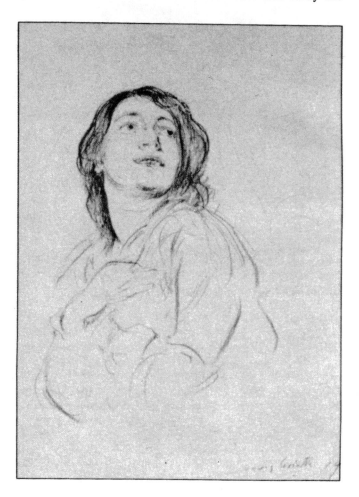

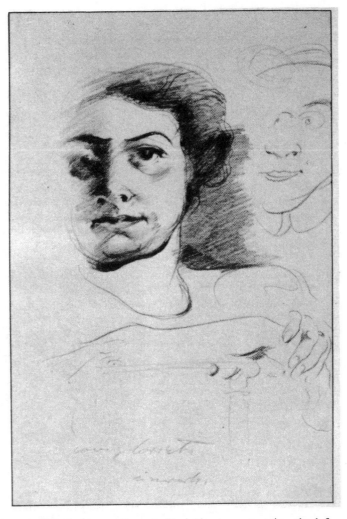

actually missing, as though Corinth was not seeing the left visual field.

I have scarcely mentioned the subjects of brain damage and disease until now because this book describes the behaviour of normal brains. Yet there is a vast literature devoted to brain pathology, and it is scarcely surprising that the research which has revealed so much about normal brain function was often undertaken with the hope that it would help doctors treat disease.

A great deal is known about diseases that reflect organic brain malfunctions, conditions like stroke, dementia, mental retardation, epilepsy and Parkinson's disease. Stroke cannot be predicted or prevented, but with proper care and retraining many patients can often regain lost functions. Dementia is a disease of the elderly though it does occur amongst younger people. It, too, is unpredictable, nor can it be stopped in most cases once the symptoms appear. Mental retardation may be prevented in infants if the causes can be identified before or immediately after birth. Sadly, in most cases the cause has not been determined even years later. As with a stroke, proper care can at least assure the afflicted individuals a comfortable life. Many epileptics need never suffer the symptoms of their disease because modern drugs can control them. Parkinsonian patients can also expect longer lives and better control over their symptoms thanks to new drugs. Yet in the main, organic brain disease can neither be prevented nor cured.

The brain disorders that more often concern both doctors and the general public, however, are the functional illnesses. These are the conditions without clearly organic causes, like anxiety, depression and schizophrenia. Unlike many of the organic disorders, these illnesses are rarely fatal, but the functional disorders affect many more people. Except for the baffling flaws in their minds, these patients often appear to be healthy and potentially productive citizens. After centuries of research and theorizing, neither the prevention nor the cure of these conditions seems to be much nearer.

In some patients, the functional diseases almost certainly do have organic causes and are, therefore, mislabelled. Evidence supporting this statement comes primarily from studies of the effects of the drugs used to control the symptoms. Thus, certain major tranquillizers are chemicals called benzodiazepines. To control anxiety, depression or schizophrenic excitement, the drugs must alter the activities of neurons somewhere. You may remember that in Chapter 6 we examined the natural opiates discovered because it was assumed that receptors for morphine must have come into existence to subserve a native body chemical. Similarly, the benzodiazepine tranquillizers link up with receptors which must have been performing some function before these drugs came along. Is there a natural tranquillizer? Again, the answer seems to be, yes. It may be that anxiety, for example, reflects either a shortage of this natural substance or some failure in the receptors for it. Even so, the diseases are probably more complex malfunctions. Depression is often associated with memories of failed love, death and bereavement or family unhappiness. Schizophrenia is said by some authorities to be caused by continuous perceptual errors. As we have seen, memory and perception are themselves grounded in physiological activities. Accordingly, the functional disorders may originate with an environmental experience which disrupts some aspect of brain chemistry. It may then be true, as psychotherapists have hoped for many years, that proper treatment of the environmental trigger can permit the physical malfunction to right itself.

Yet nothing has been done to reduce the numbers of the mentally ill. They occupy one-fifth of all hospital beds in the United Kingdom and the United States. As much as half the time of general practitioners must be devoted to reassuring patients whose troubles are not obviously physical. The GP often performs functions once left to the family or the priest. Britain's general practitioners issue more prescriptions for Valium and Librium than for all other prescription drugs combined.

Both because it has been around longer and because it is used to treat far more people than drugs or shock therapy, psychotherapy has borne the brunt of mental medicine. It has failed and still fails to stay the flood. H. J. Eysenck, the British psychiatrist, studied a larger number of psychiatric patients and found that about 75 per cent who entered psychotherapy improved or recovered. That is hardly failure, but Eysenck also discovered that of those patients who complained to their GPs but had received no psychotherapeutic treatment, about 75 per cent also improved or recovered! There is no evidence that any form of psychotherapy consistently helps patients. The best that can be said is that thousands of unhappy people can share their problems with professionally-trained people who may be able to mitigate the loneliness or fear of their patients.

One reason for the unsatisfactory record of psychotherapy is that diagnosis is extremely uncertain. Without clear physical signs, the physician is forced to interpret subjective symptoms which are often disjointed and contradictory.

In the early 1970s an American professor of psychology, D. L. Rosenhan, got seven friends and associates to join him in an experiment. Three were women, and all but one was over thirty. They included a pediatrician, a painter, a housewife and five psychologists. All were legally and socially sane. The object of the experiment was to demonstrate the inadequacy of diagnosis.

Despite their undeniable health, all eight subjects set out to obtain admission to twelve mental hospitals in five states. Of the twelve, one was a private hospital, one was supported by a university and ten were public institutions. Obviously, some of the subjects were admitted to more than one institution. At each hospital the pseudo-patient rang for an appointment. Each used a pseudonym, and the psychologists also gave false occupations. All other biographical details were truthful except one: each patient described a symptom which had been agreed to in advance by the subjects. Each patient had heard voices. The voices spoke unclearly and were unfamiliar, but they were of the same sex as the pseudo-patient. This symptom was chosen because it is reasonably straightforward and is 'alleged to arise from painful concerns about the perceived meaninglessness of one's life'. All twelve applications for admission were accepted.

Eleven were diagnosed as schizophrenic and the twelfth as manic-depressive psychotic. The twelve spent between seven and fifty-two days in hospital with an average stay of nine-teen days. Once they were admitted, the pseudo-patients heard no more voices. Their behaviour was exemplary. None knew when he or she would be discharged, but they had no wish to remain in the mental wards any longer than they had to.

They all kept notes of the details of their treatments and surroundings. At first they tried to hide their journals, but the staff ignored their notetaking so that concealment seemed pointless. They accepted drugs, but disposed of them. Doctors appeared on the wards about seven times each day on average. Nurses averaged about 11 per cent of their time mingling with patients. The balance of their shifts were spent in staff areas. The pseudo-patients approached thirteen doctors and forty-seven nurses with polite questions about their conditions. There were 185 such approaches to doctors and 1285 to other staff, the over-whelming majority of which were absolutely ignored. In the hospital records there are no complaints against any of the pseudo-patients.

No hospital questioned the simulation. Yet 35 per cent of 188 real patients on whom notes were kept during the first three hospitalizations stated that they thought the pseudo-patients were fakes. All eleven 'schizophrenics' were released with the diagnosis 'schizophrenia in remission', a common experience for about half of all real schizophrenics. 'It is clear,' Dr Rosenhan concluded, 'that we cannot distin-guish the sane from the insane in psychiatric hospitals.'

Schizophrenia is a severe personality disturbance with symptoms which often cause the patient great pain and disablement. If such a serious disease can be mistaken, what about the diagnosis of the patient who is anxious or depressed? Anxiety and depression are feelings we all experi-ence occasionally. In theory we are not ill until we are unable to carry on a normal life. Yet the ability to cope is apparently a pretty shifting platform. There is probably no one reading this book who has not sometimes felt: I just can't cope for another minute.

Death, it has been observed, is nature's way of telling you to slow down. Life, on the other hand, is one long problem. Nor is that hyperbole. If you look at it from the standpoint of the great French physiologist, Claude Bernard, every organism seeks to maintain itself in the face of baleful nature. Homeostasis requires adaptability and effort, as we noted in Chapter 3. The notion that life is a mere pilgrimage through a vale of tears has considerable biological sanction.

Yet most of us get on with it and experience a certain amount of satisfaction in the process. Perhaps the supreme role of the brain is to help its owner meet and overcome strains and stresses.

Are you lonely, for example? Why? Have you accepted a situation that only you can change?

Is your sex life unsatisfactory? You alone can correct that, too. Are you allowing superstition or prejudice to stand in your way?

Unemployed? This disaster is certainly not of your making, at least not in most cases. But is there nothing at all for you to do? No garden, children, car, house – nothing needing your attention? Have you offered your help to a political party or trade union trying to correct the causes of unemployment?

Bereaved? You know that death is inevitable. Even if it was premature, you are alive. Can you not wash your face, tidy your kitchen, eat a meal, talk to willing friends – spend a little of the small change of life?

Unless you are really ill, you must eventually help yourself. Even when you cannot and feel that you must have help, then only you can see your doctor. Just the effort may help you as much as he can. In the present state of the psychotherapeutic art, you may be the best doctor for your own anxiety or depression.

Look at your problem as squarely as you can. Your dreams may help your understanding. Perhaps by facing up to things, edges will begin to chip away so that you can begin to see around the boulders in your way. Often there is more than one path. Just try not to sit alone suffering. Try to act. After all, real illness is much less common than normal health, and the odds are that you are as competent at living as anyone. You have made it this far.

Just one caveat. Please do not think that the opposite of mental illness is happiness. Happiness may be a new puppy when you are ten years old, or the feeling when you know your love is reciprocated, but it is not for everyday. I think one of the most mischievous myths of modern life sets happiness as the goal. Toothpaste and hi-fi may bring enjoyment, even satisfaction – but happiness? Like the excitement of discovery, the joy of music, happiness happens occasionally, unexpectedly. Surely, most of the time we must accept just getting on and let the miracles take care of themselves. Mental health belongs to most of us merely because we change the diapers, drive the buses, type the letters, mind the computers and study the world or the bodies we live in – all of life's ordinary brain games. That is the great thing about health. You get it by doing something else.

Game 10.2, continued: At least a week should have passed before you finish this game. Do not look at your previous analysis yet. Study the Rorschach-type ink blot again, and again write down what you see. Now, compare this analysis to the earlier one. If there are differences, can you explain them? Do you think this book has helped you to explain the differences? At the least, I hope that your explanation of this and other changes in your mental life will seem less mysterious than they were before you played these *Brain Games*.

Glossary

Action potential. The flow of postively-charged *ions* into a *neuron* which suddenly and briefly reverses the charge difference between the exterior and interior of the cell. The neuronal signal.

Adaptation. Psychological perception of neuronal 'tiring', leading to temporary loss of sensation from the *neurons* involved. By comparison, habituation is loss of perception due to inattention. Adaptability is a characteristic of organisms permitting them to continue to live in any given environment.

Axon. Process of a *neuron* along which the *action potential* normally moves from the cell body to the axon bulb where *transmitter* may be released. The axon branches infrequently if at all and tends to retain its thickness throughout its length. Lengths vary from a few mms to a meter. Some axons are myelinated (see *myelin*).

Cerebellum. Little brain. The part of the brain above the hind-brain and beneath the *occipital* lobes which regulates fine movement.

Chunking. The technique of grouping information to increase the amount perceived and remembered; for example, rhythmic chunking of sounds, chunking of letters into words.

Cochlea. The bony spiral of the inner ear containing the organ of sound sensing.

Colliculus. One of four small protuberances on top of the hind-brain grouped in twos as the superior (upper) and inferior (lower) colliculi. The colliculi receive touch, aural and visual sensation, and in the human brain regulate attention.

Conditioning. A learning technique in which a response to a stimulus is redirected to some other stimulus. In classical conditioning, as introduced by the Russian physiologist, I. P. Pavlov, the subject has no influence over the conditioning but learns to transfer an unconditioned response to some new stimulus. In operant conditioning, introduced by the American psychologist, B. F. Skinner, the subject can alter the stimulus by changing its response.

Continuum. An infinite series of points forming an imaginary straight line connecting extremes. In psychology, the opposite is discontinuous; i.e., a series of discrete but related finite traits.

Corpus callosum. The mass of myelinated (see *myelin*) *axons* linking the two hemispheres of the cerebral *cortex.*

Cortex. Any outer layer of tissue surrounding other layers; thus, the adrenal cortex. The largest part of the human brain with a characteristically coruscated surface hiding the mid- and hind-brain and the cerebellum. The cortex grew out of the olfactory bulb and is the newest part of the brain from the evolutionary standpoint. It receives sensations and regulates voluntary and some involuntary movement and is probably the site of memory, learned emotion and perception.

Dendrite. Process of a *neuron* which receives signals from other neurons. Except in neurons the dendrites of which are specialized to receive sensations, dendrites are usually densely arborized with the branches thinning towards their tips.

Drive. In psychology, a motivation, that expression of the self which produces behaviour.

Electroencephalogram (EEG). Recording either permanently in ink on a moving paper drum or in temporary visual display on an oscilloscope of the electrical activity in the brain beneath electrodes placed on the hair or scalp.

Excitability. A physical quality of *neurons* and muscle cells which causes these cells to react to suitable stimulation by a reversible change in cell state.

Excitatory. The induction of *excitability*. Thus, a *neuron* and a *transmitter* may be either excitatory or inhibitory. An inhibitory neuron or transmitter reduces the excitability of the next post-synaptic (see *synapse*) neuron.

Extroversion. One extreme in a *continuum,* extroversion-introversion, describing a personality trait. Extroversion means turning one's interest and attention outside oneself. Introversion means turning one's interest and attention on to oneself.

Ganglion. A junction formed by several *neurons* consisting of *synapses* between *axon* bulbs and *dendrites* or cell bodies. The brain is the largest ganglion.

Glial cell. The non-nervous, non-excitable (see *excitability*) brain cells which insulate *neurons* and assist in their nutrition and support.

Gyrus. A curved mound of brain tissue, usually longer than it is wide, observed on the surface of the *cortex* between *sulci.*

Habituation. See *Adaptation.*

Hippocampus. A bilateral centre in the mid-brain consisting of regular neuronal arrays thought to be involved in the formation of long-term spatial memory. (Lit.: see monster.)

Homeostasis. The tendency of living things to achieve balance or stability. Introduced in this meaning by the American physiologist, W. B. Cannon.

Hormone. A chemical secreted into the blood which acts on cells elsewhere in the body to produce a physiological effect.

Hypothalamus. A bilateral centre in the mid-brain consisting of many neuronal nuclei with functions affecting emotions of fear, pleasure and anger, the hunger and thirst *drives*, temperature regulation and the secretion of several *hormones* known as *releasing factors.*

Inhibitory. See *Excitatory.*

Intelligence quotient (*IQ*). One's score on an intelligence test placing one in relation to others within the same group however defined.

Introversion. See *Extroversion.*

Ion. An electrically-charged atom or group of atoms.

Lateralization. The specialization of one side of the brain to regulate certain functions more or less exclusively. Not to be confused with laterality – left- or right-handedness, or with the tendency of the right side of the brain to regulate sensation and movement in the left side of the body and vice versa. Lateralization is usually applied to language functions which are regulated in most people by the left cortical hemisphere.

Microelectrode. An electrode miniaturized so that its point can be placed beside or inside a single cell.

Millisecond. One thousandth (0.001) of a second.

Motivation. See *Drive.*

Myelin. A fat-like chemical synthesized by certain *glial* cells to form a layered white insulation around the *axons* of some *neurons.* White matter consists of large numbers of myelinated axons.

Nerve. See *Neuron.*

Neuron. A nerve cell. A nerve, however, consists of several neurons. Each neuron or the *axon* of each neuron in a nerve is sometimes called a nerve fibre. Nerves are often visible to the naked eye, especially if the axons are myelinated (see *myelin*).

Occipital. The bilateral rear lobes of the *cortex.*

Parameter. An identifying quality that individuals share with one another which can be kept constant while other qualities may be varied.

Parietal. Bilateral upper central lobes of *cortex.*

Pathway. A temporary or permanent sequence of *neurons* which has a physiological or a psychological function.

Quotient. See *Intelligence quotient.*

Receptor. A molecule or molecular group in a cell which chemically binds other molecules thereby leading to some change in cell function.

Releasing factor. A hypothalamic (see *hypothalamus*) *hormone* stimulating synthesis of a pituitary hormone.

Reticular activating system. Also Reticular formation. A network (reticulum) of *neurons* linking mid- and hind-brain and so intimately interlinked that waves of excitation move through it. Thus, it serves to activate or awaken the organism.

Sulcus. The valleys in the *cortex* forming the gyri (see *gyrus*).

Synapse. The near juxtaposition of an *axon* bulb and a dendrite or cell body. The space itself is called the synaptic gap.

Temporal. Bilateral lower central lobes of the *cortex*.

Thalamus. Bilateral mid-brain relay centre for sensory data and motor signals.

Transmitter. A chemical released at the *axon* bulb of a signalling *neuron* so that it diffuses across the *synapse* to *receptors* on a post-synaptic neuron causing changes in the chemical properties of the latter. The trans-synaptic or interneuronal signal.

Vestibulary system. Bilateral organ of balance in the inner ear.

References

CHAPTER 1

Game 1.1: Based on Stanley Coren, Clare Porac, Lawrence M. Ward, *Sensation and Perception* (New York, San Francisco, London, Academic Press, 1979), p. 420

Game 1.3: John Nicholson, *A Question of Sex* (London, Fontana, 1979), p. 93

Game 1.5: Nicholson, *Sex*, pp. 87–8

Game 1.8: Adapted from Nicholson, *Sex*, pp. 17–18

Game 1.9: Ronald Forgus and B. H. Shulman, *Personality: A Cognitive View* (Englewood Cliffs, N.J., Prentice-Hall, 1979), p. 282

Game 1.10: Robert Gottsdanker, *Experimenting in Psychology* (Englewood Cliffs, N.J., Prentice-Hall, 1978), p. 310

Game 1.11: Forgus and Shulman, *Personality*, pp. 4–5

CHAPTER 2

Game 2.1: Keith Oatley, *Brain Mechanisms and Mind* (New York, Dutton, 1973), p. 65

A. R. Luria, *The Man with a Shattered World* (New York, Basic Books, 1972)

CHAPTER 3

Solomon's puppies: John Brierley, *The Thinking Machine* (Wayne, N.J., Fairleigh Dickinson, 1973), p. 82

Formula for consciousness: Steven Rose, *The Conscious Brain* (New York, Random House, 1976), p. 144

'Self-esteem': William James, *Psychology* (Cleveland and New York, Modern Library, 1948), p. 187

J. E. LeDoux, D. H. Wilson and M. S. Gazzaniga: 'Beyond Commissurotomy: Clues to Consciousness', *Handbook of Behavioral Neurobiology*, Vol 2, *Neuropsychology*, edited by M. S. Gazzaniga (New York and London, Plenum, 1979), p. 550

CHAPTER 4

Game 4.1: Max Wertheimer, *Productive Thinking,* edited by Michael Wertheimer (New York, Greenwood, 1978), pp. 143–144

Game 4.3: Wertheimer, *Productive Thinking*, p. 123

Game 4.5: A. R. Luria, *The Making of Mind: A Personal Account of Soviet Psychology*, edited by M. and S. Cole (Cambridge, Mass., and London, Harvard University Press, 1979), pp. 72–3

Games 4.6–4.9: Norman Sullivan, *Use Your Intelligence* (London, Fontana, 1978), pp. 25–8. Illustration by David Woodroffe.

Divergent questions: Lee J. Cronbach, *Essentials of Psychological Testing* (New York, Evanston and London, Harper and Row, 1970), pp. 336 ff.

Game 4.12: My thanks to Derek and Julia Parker, authors of *How Do You Know Who You Are?* (New York, Macmillan, 1980), who were most helpful with this game.

CHAPTER 5

Rose: *Conscious Brain*, p. 190

Anthony Storr: *The Art of Psychotherapy* (New York, Methuen, 1980), p. 24

A. R. Luria: *The Mind of a Mnemonist* (Chicago, Contemporary, 1968)

Game 5.19: Peter Russell, *The Brain Book* (New York, Dutton, 1979), p. 126

Young's model: Rose, *Conscious Brain,* p. 210

CHAPTER 6

Jean Piaget: *Origins of Intelligence in Children* (New York, International Universities Press, 1952), p. 335; quoted in Peter H. Lindsay and Donald A. Norman, *Human Information Processing: An Introduction to Psychology* (New York and London, Academic Press, 1972), pp. 488–9

Herbert S. Terrace: *Nim* (New York, Knopf, 1979)

Phrase structure rules: Roger Brown, and Richard J. Herrnstein, *Psychology* (Boston, Little, Brown, 1975), pp. 452–3

Computer-human conversation: Lindsay and Norman, *Human Information Processing*, p. 382

'Tie knots': A.R. Luria, *The Working Brain: An Introduction to Neuropsychology* (New York, Basic Books, 1973), p. 31

'Motor automatism': Luria, *Working Brain*, p. 140

CHAPTER 7

Vernon Mountcastle: cited in Steven Rose, *Conscious Brain*, p. 101

Helen Keller: *The Story of My Life* (New York, Doubleday, 1931), pp. 21–2; quoted in Coren *et al.*, *Sensation*, p. 116

Game 7.6: Coren *et al.*, *Sensation*, p. 234

Game 7.7: Idem.

Game 7.8 and diagram: Coren *et al.*, *Sensation*, p. 127

Game 7.9 and diagram: Coren *et al.*, *Sensation*, p. 232

Ronald Melzack: *The Puzzle of Pain* (New York, Basic Books, 1973)

Game 7.14: Coren *et al.*, *Sensation*, p. 135

Game 7.16: Coren *et al.*, *Sensation*, p. 99

Game 7.18: Coren *et al.*, *Sensation*, p. 106

CHAPTER 8

Game 8.1: Coren *et al.*, *Sensation*, p. 66

Game 8.5: Coren *et al.*, *Sensation*, p. 72

Game 8.6: Coren *et al.*, *Sensation*, p. 159
Game 8.8: Coren *et al.*, *Sensation*, p. 291
Game 8.10: John P. Frisby, *Seeing: Illusion, Brain and Mind* (Oxford, New York, Toronto, Melbourne, Oxford University Press, 1979), p. 139
Game 8.1: Frisby, *Seeing*, p. 92
Game 8.12: Frisby, *Seeing*, p. 93
Game 8.13: Frisby, *Seeing*, p. 98
Tilt after effect: Frisby, *Seeing*, p. 99
'Happy to live with a paradox': Frisby, *Seeing*, p. 101
Game 8.15: Frisby, *Seeing*, p. 124
Game 8.16: Frisby, *Seeing*, p. 125
Game 8.17: Coren *et al.*, *Sensation*, p. 259

CHAPTER 10

Richard Gregory, *The Intelligent Eye* (New York, McGraw Hill, 1970), p. 31
Luria: *Making of Mind,* p. 80
Game 10.2: George A. Miller, *Psychology, the Science of Mental Life* (New York, Harper & Row, 1973), p. 57
Game 10.3: Coren *et al.*, *Sensation*, p. 413
Game 10.4: Coren *et al.*, *Sensation*, p. 415
Game 10.6: Lindsay and Norman, *Human Information Processing*, p. 8
Game 10.7: Oatley, *Brain Mechanisms*, p. 19
Proximity: Miller, *Psychology*, p. 142
Similarity: Miller, *Psychology*, p. 143
Game 10.8: Coren *et al.*, *Sensation*, p. 309
Gregory, *Intelligent Eye*, p. 120
Game 10.9: Miller, *Psychology*, p. 130
Game 10.10: Lindsay and Norman, *Human Information Processing*, p. 134
Game 10.15: Lindsay and Norman, *Human Information Processing*, p. 15
Game 10.17: Coren *et al.*, *Sensation*, p. 283
Games 10.20, 10.21: Brown and Herrnstein, *Psychology*, p. 382

Colour charts: Coren *et al.*, *Sensation*, p. 171
Game 10.25: Coren *et al.*, *Sensation*, p. 289
Game 10.29: Coren *et al.* *Sensation*, p. 405
Game 10.30: Coren *et al.*, *Sensation*, p. 37
Game 10.31: Lindsay and Norman, *Human Information Processing*, p. 135
Pandemonium: based on Lindsay and Norman, *Human Information Processing*, p. 121

AFTERWORD

D. L. Rosenhan: 'On being sane in insane places', *Science*, 179 (1973), pp. 250–8

Further Reading

The most important sources for the ideas in the *Manual* are listed in the References. Of these items, three books are both entertaining and full of up-to-the-minute information.

Stanley Coren, Clare Porac, Lawrence M. Ward, *Sensation and Perception* (New York, San Francisco, London, Academic Press, 1979), is a textbook published in a paperback edition.

Peter H. Lindsay and Donald A. Norman, *Human Information Processing: An Introduction to Psychology* (New York and London, Academic Press, 1972), is also published in a paperback edition.

Neither book is cheap, but both are well illustrated and display a welcome absence of intellectual stuffiness.

John P. Frisby, *Seeing: Illusion, Brain and Mind* (Oxford, New York, Toronto, Melbourne, Oxford University Press, 1979), has been published only in hardcover. It explores some of the same ground as Coren *et al.*, and offers precise insights into the connection between psychological perception and the physiological activities of some neurons.

Any book by the Russian neuropsychologist, A. R. Luria, is worth reading. Four are listed under References, but his most general statement in English is *The Working Brain: An Introduction to Neuropsychology* (New York, Basic Books, 1973).

Many other popular introductions to brain function have been published. The interested reader must approach each one with care because even professional scientists can become unstuck when they confront the need to explain the brain. Speculation seems to be justified by the grandeur of the subject if not by the hard data actually available. The reader must approach every claim with skepticism. If you are always doubtful, you are unlikely to be swept up by some imaginative but insubstantial notion, for example, that all your problems can be solved by deep breathing. Books about the brain are especially prone to this kind of idiocy and must be read with appropriate caution.

Index

Index